Managing Uncertainty in Mental Health Care

Managing Uncertainty in Mental Health Care

José Silveira, MD, BSc, FRCPC

Associate Professor
Department of Psychiatry
University of Toronto
Toronto, ON, Canada

Patricia Rockman, HBA, MD, CCFP

Associate Professor
Department of Family and Community Medicine Cross-Appointed to Psychiatry
University of Toronto
Toronto, ON, Canada

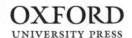

OXFORD
UNIVERSITY PRESS

OXFORD
UNIVERSITY PRESS

Oxford University Press is a department of the University of Oxford. It furthers
the University's objective of excellence in research, scholarship, and education
by publishing worldwide. Oxford is a registered trade mark of Oxford University
Press in the UK and certain other countries.

Published in the United States of America by Oxford University Press
198 Madison Avenue, New York, NY 10016, United States of America.

Library of Congress Cataloging-in-Publication Data
Names: Silveira, José (Psychiatrist) author. | Rockman, Patricia, author.
Title: Managing uncertainty in mental health care /
by José Silveira and Patricia Rockman.
Description: New York, NY : Oxford University Press, [2021] |
Includes bibliographical references and index.
Identifiers: LCCN 2021032310 (print) | LCCN 2021032311 (ebook) |
ISBN 9780197509326 (paperback) |
ISBN 9780197509340 (epub) | ISBN 9780197509357 (digital online)
Subjects: MESH: Mental Disorders—diagnosis |
Clinical Decision-Making | Uncertainty
Classification: LCC RC469 (print) | LCC RC469 (ebook) |
NLM WM 141 | DDC 616.89/075—dc23
LC record available at https://lccn.loc.gov/2021032310
LC ebook record available at https://lccn.loc.gov/2021032311

DOI: 10.1093/med/9780197509326.001.0001

1 3 5 7 9 8 6 4 2
Printed by Marquis, Canada

For Salomé and José
—JS

For Casey Fulford, to assist her on her journey.
—PR

Contents

Acknowledgments

From José: I would like to thank my spouse Flora Ricciuti and my son Zachary for tolerating my indulgence.

From Patricia: To Bryan Moran, my life partner, for his emotional and financial support during the writing of this book.

We also thank Pat Croskerry, Anthony King, Evan Collins, Michael Cheng, Mireille St.-Jean, Daniel McBain and Ryan Kamstra for reviewing, editing, and commenting on the manuscript.

Conversations with the following people were extremely helpful to the creation of this work: Mark Zimmerman, Gustavo Saposnik, Lee Freedman, and Casey Fulford. Jon Hunter, a dear colleague, supported and encouraged us frequently along the way, when others were dismissive of the concepts.

The Centre for Effective Practice, the Ontario College of Family Physicians Collaborative Mental Health Care Network, the University of Toronto, Department of Family and Community Medicine, and the Canadian Family Physician provided us with a variety of platforms to develop the ideas in this book.

Last, we express our appreciation to Andrea Knobloch at Oxford University Press for allowing us this opportunity.

Introduction

The shortest distance between two points is a straight line. The trick is to figure out if they should be connected and whether a straight line is applicable. This is what this book is about, the hidden and enigmatic uncertainty inherent to mental health and addictions, which is often disguised as the familiar and the simple in clinical practice. It is also about us, clinicians, struggling to help people drowning in their distress and who sometimes draw others down with them. Regardless of the discipline in which we work or our level of expertise, we all face the same irreducible uncertainty when managing mental disorders. We are not unlike meteorologists, wrestling with nature's chaos to make pronouncements.

Like meteorologists, clinicians try to impose order on the disorder, often creating narratives that are incomplete or wrong. The illumination intended by our nosology and current knowledge fades quickly as we apply it to the complexity of our domain. We are nonetheless expected to make judgments and decisions, often while negotiating competing demands.

As clinicians, we treat individuals. Of course, individuals belong to populations, but each person experiences a unique journey that shapes their brain and mind into one of a kind. Each person, therefore, deviates from the script written from population studies with problems and treatment responses not addressed in the available knowledge.

In addition to the gaps in our knowledge and the limits of available clinical methods, we face a third challenge—the human mind's automatic response to objective uncertainty. Ironically, our mind's solution is unwarranted certainty and overconfidence. Our aim is to weave all three challenges into a compelling narrative with a novel perspective on the challenges clinicians face and how we might meet them. This picture may leave you incredulous at times but, hopefully, also compassionate toward yourself. We also hope you will be less quick to regard your errors as unique to you and that this will help you shed unwarranted confidence and certainty in your judgments and decisions.

Why Focus on Uncertainty?

Although our book focuses on objective uncertainty in mental health and addictions, the discussion and concepts are relevant to any clinical area.

Mental disorders simply warrant more direct attention because of the absence of known etiologies, pathophysiology, or objective measures. Nonetheless, the enormous impact of these conditions requires our attention.

Despite the degree of complexity, ambiguity, and inadequate collective knowledge, most clinicians rarely experience subjective uncertainty in daily practice. In the rare instances that anyone fully appreciates the enigmas confronting them, the discomfort of not knowing is unsettling. Clinicians, however, have the added discomfort of being formally accountable to others for the judgments we make. Uncertainty is this book's focus because we recognize the clinician's challenge in making clairvoyant decisions about the future based on opaque views of the past and an often blurry present. Clinicians managing mental disorders are dependent on crude knowledge, incomplete information, and an absence of clear and consistent outcome measures.

Even the most basic terminology used in the area of mental health is a moving target rife with controversy. Most notably, this is reflected in the debate of whether we are referring to disorders of brain, mind, or spirit. This quarrel has carried on for centuries with no resolution. The bulk of this controversy is fuelled by cultural values and beliefs that insufficient science has been unable to correct. We humbly accept that all views have an equal probability of being wrong and believe the disagreement in terminology reflects the depth to which uncertainty challenges us all—communities, researchers, and clinicians alike.

Our families, friends, and coworkers cannot wait for us to resolve these theoretical controversies. We discuss emerging transdiagnostic approaches to guide assessment while accounting for the enigmatic nature of mental health. Our aim is to chart a course using an approach to risk, functional impairments, and relevant symptoms, to reduce harm, enhance function, and reduce suffering.

Assessment and identification of risk can be particularly difficult due to the unknowns in undifferentiated presentations. This book addresses the utility of our nosology, the rampant issue of diagnostic error, and suggests approaches for dealing with the lack of predictability that is often deemphasized in clinical practice. It is, in the final analysis, a call for an adoption of pragmatic humility.

Last, respecting the healthy debate about labels, we have chosen to use the term *patient* to denote the role delineation that occurs when a person in society interacts, by necessity, with a health care system. Elsewhere, we have used the words person, people, or client.

1

Uncertainty and the Certainty Bias

> The need for certainty is the greatest disease the mind faces.
> —Robert Greene

The Certainty Bias

The degree of complexity of the brain, mind, and the environments in which humans live would predict that mental health clinicians work in a perpetual state of uncertainty. That prediction would be wrong. To the contrary, in clinical practice, our brains exhibit the same pedestrian bias toward irrational certainty.[1-5] Given the degree of complexity in the field of mental health, it is remarkable that we clinicians can assist anyone at all.

Our professional training ratifies the scientific method in an attempt to protect us and those we treat from unwarranted certainty. Current training, however, appears to be inadequate to this task. The assessment and management of mental disorders, across specialists and nonspecialists alike, is associated with ubiquitous feelings of certainty. Feeling certain despite the degree of inherent complexity and ambiguity. Feeling certain despite the rudimentary state of empirical knowledge. Feeling certain despite the absence of technologically objective methods to assist assessment or evaluate treatment results.

Clinicians are not alone. All humans are afflicted with a set of peculiar tendencies in perceiving and thinking that, collectively, create an illusion that our judgments and beliefs are correct. These tendencies can be listed as the certainty bias, the overconfidence bias, and the optimism bias. Whether they are different aspects of the mind's attempt to negotiate the unpredictable complexity of the world is less relevant than the view that each perspective gives us into our response to uncertainty. The power of this illusion's hold on our minds is impressive. It is resistant to a range of professional training methods in multiple disciplines. It is also resistant to experience. After years of rigorous training and practice, psychologists, psychiatrists, financial analysts, physicians, and others still can't check their overconfidence. Unwarranted certainty consistently emerges in judgment and action. From the perspective of this immutability, unwarranted certainty acts upon us more like an illusion than a cognitive error. It seems to be a default position of the mind—one that is considerably more pleasant to accept than question.[2] It is not, however, intentional or benign.

The repercussions of the certainty bias on clinician effectiveness are prodigious and are detailed in Chapters 5 and 6. These repercussions are also surprising given the extent to which unwarranted certainty is neglected in training and practice. Its presence fuels premature diagnostic closure and other cognitive biases that lead to errors of judgment and decision.[6]

When uncertainty is formally acknowledged, it is discussed in a manner that suggests it is a greater evil than certainty. This is in the form of arguments that certainty allows us to cut through complexity to enable acting when urgently required. This argument, however, ignores the ensuing failures and that acknowledging uncertainty promotes reconsideration of whether our actions were appropriate. Without subjective uncertainty to prompt such reflection, clinicians fail to learn from experience. So, although we frequently act under the pressure of limited time, unwarranted certainty is neither necessary nor an advantage in responding urgently. Acknowledging the uncertainty in our work is essential to providing optimal care and translating clinical experience into improved performance.

Another area of concern in the literature is that clinician uncertainty may result in a phenomenon known as *therapeutic inertia*. This concept refers to a hesitation to initiate appropriate treatment or failure to alter it despite an absence of progress.[7-9] This is well studied in numerous areas of medicine other than in the treatment of mental disorders.[10-15] The extent to which perceived uncertainty contributes to therapeutic inertia, however, is likely to be minimal. Clinicians do not experience significant doubt in their judgments and decisions. So, although therapeutic inertia may be a useful concept to consider in quality improvement, its primary antecedents do not arise from subjective uncertainty.

Uncertainty is also inherent to the very research findings that form our knowledge base and shape our judgments. Unfortunately, theories and even *facts* prove to be temporary. Fortunately, contemporary research cautions that we maintain skepticism about findings in group-level data by clearly stating the probability of error using confidence intervals and other statistical techniques. Even when group-level data are solid, it does not ease the challenge of applying this information to individuals where objective uncertainty in assessment and interventions is greatest.[8-11,14]

This book is about coming to grips with the uncertainty inherent to the assessment of people presenting with possible mental disorders. It is an exploration of the impact of objective uncertainty on clinical judgment and decision making and its relevance to mental health care. This is independent of the clinical context and practitioner's professional affiliation. Last, it is about developing a transdiagnostic approach to mitigating errors of judgment. This is especially important when attempting to identify risks of harm, functional impairments, and symptoms of distress. The aim is to facilitate interventions despite diagnostic ambiguity. This is not to eschew the use of diagnostic categories to organize one's thinking. It is, however, an argument for incorporating the limitations of nosologies and related assessment methods into clinical approaches. To date, clinical approaches have been predicated upon the assumption that our nosology is valid (vis-à-vis nature), accurate, unambiguous, and thus free of error, as long as clinicians are competent. Evidence related to assessment error in mental health care, however, suggests otherwise. We need to shift to approaches that are designed with clinician errors in mind rather than pretending that irreducible uncertainty and inevitable error are insignificant.

During the past decade, we have developed a transdiagnostic approach to managing uncertainty and its antecedents in our domain. During this period, we have encountered both acceptance and opposition to it within family medicine, social work, psychology, and psychiatry. This is consistent with controversies occurring more broadly in mental health. Leaders in nosology have been questioning the validity and effectiveness of diagnostic constructs in facilitating the understanding of psychopathology and its treatment. From these robust debates have emerged cogent arguments for mental health to incorporate more phenomenologically based approaches in research and practice.[16,17]

In addition, we question the field's reliance on the patient's story as the authoritative source of information for accurate assessments. At the best of times, the coherence of the human narrative and explanations for our behavior and emotions are often inaccurate. The idea that an unstructured narrative framework and explanatory models have limitations has also evoked both support and denigration. We are encouraged by thoughtful experts who have also identified this reliance as one of the barriers to improving our success in addressing mental disorders.[18]

Given the absence of clarity related to managing people with mental disorders, why do we clinicians tend to be so confident in our judgments and decisions? Why is it that we do not acknowledge objective uncertainty with greater frequency, whether it's in the literature or with our colleagues

and patients? Why are we not educated to prioritize it as a factor that significantly constrains the accuracy of our judgments and fuels clinical error, independent of competence? It is interesting how much we support our sense of
certainty with the notion of "evidence-based practice" despite the mutability
of research findings. It's as if evidence has become the destination rather than
milestones on our journey. Can we embrace uncertainty and even use it as a
guide to our clinical advantage?

To address these questions requires awareness of the fascinating predilection of humans for certainty and our ubiquitous discomfort with its absence.

The Discomfort with Uncertainty

Let's begin with our discomfort with uncertainty. Upon reflection, most of
us recognize that uncertainty triggers anxiety. As the neurologist Gustavo
Saposnik states, "Most physicians must make diagnostic and therapeutic
decisions under uncertainty with insufficient or imperfect information. As
such, individual physicians' tolerance to uncertainty may affect decisions in
clinical care."[19]

Clinicians are not educated and trained to identify and manage uncertainty.
We are, ostensibly, socialized to initially hypothesize but ultimately to know.
You don't get kudos in professional training for saying "I don't know" or "I'm
not sure." The student is not socialized to openly question axioms or bring a
beginner's mind to a clinical situation. Rather, they are acculturated to believe
that what they are learning is immutable rather than evolving, and contingent.
This is perpetuated throughout our careers. This may be an effective approach
to reduce anxiety and enable professions to project authority and expertise. Problems arise, however, when this framework shapes the judgment of
clinicians treating people with complex and ambiguous conditions that defy
precision. We will explore this more completely to illustrate the extent of our
discomfort with uncertainty, the problems associated with avoiding it, and investigate our habitual tendencies when faced with it.

The bias toward certainty tends to go unrecognized, and any related anxiety, even if acknowledged, is quickly buried by minimizing the implications
of uncertainty.[20,21] Uncertainty and anxiety can be tightly bound and easily
conflated. Therefore, both the anxiety elicited and the resultant denial of the
uncertainty need to be acknowledged.

One of the negative consequences of the certainty bias is that it constricts
clinician thinking acutely and, as conditions unfold, blinds us to cues that our
impressions may be wrong or incomplete. This is especially debilitating in the

case of mental health and addictions because of the pervasive ambiguity, extensive symptom overlaps, absence of objective tests, and tendency of these disorders to declare themselves over time. We also suggest that we don't address these issues sufficiently, as is evidenced by the meager attention they receive in our training, in clinical practice, and in the literature. Acknowledging and accepting the existence of both our uncertainty and our anxiety potentially enables us to engage in adaptive strategies rather than avoidance and blind certainty. This may in turn allow us to respond to those we serve more comfortably and skillfully. Since uncertainty is certain, we may as well accept it, develop greater comfort with it, and leverage its utility.

Defining Uncertainty

What exactly is uncertainty and where does it come from? How can we define it? This is tricky given the range of definitions of uncertainty in such disciplines as psychology, clinical medicine, cognitive science, physics, statistics, and complexity science.

We provide a pragmatic definition of uncertainty that is applicable to clinical practice without ignoring the robust facets of uncertainty that make it impossible to escape. For our purposes, we limit the discussion of theoretical aspects of uncertainty to those having significant implications for clinical care.

Uncertainty did not become a medical subject heading until 2003 (United States National Library of Medicine). It is defined as "the condition in which reasonable knowledge regarding risks, benefits or the future is not available."[22] In case you missed it, let us point out that this definition does not appear to include uncertainty related to history taking, definition of phenomena, diagnosis, and other key elements in clinical practice. It is a typical definition of uncertainty in that it is future oriented. Consequently, so far as this book is concerned, the definition is insufficient for our purposes. So, let's keep searching (if you will).

A common, and pithy, definition of uncertainty refers to it as the probability of error in predictions. According to this definition, the greater the probability of error in any given prediction, the greater the uncertainty. Implicit is that uncertainty relates to the impact of multiple factors influencing the probability of error in predicting future events. However, most clinical challenges do not involve predictions. Instead, our primary tasks demand an accurate recognition of complex, evolving patterns using incomplete information that may or may not be relevant to the concern at hand. In mental health, we have the additional issue of delineating patterns related to the enigmatic brain and mind.

We also have the concept of uncertainty as it applies to the scientific or formal knowledge we utilize in our judgments and decision making. This way of thinking about uncertainty defines and deconstructs it by its sources (e.g., inside the clinician, inside the patient, inside organizational structures, or in the body of knowledge itself) and to relationships between these temporally and to us as clinicians.[23]

Our aim is to define uncertainty within the clinical context and steer us away from a deeper philosophical conversation of whether all things are knowable given enough time. The reality for clinicians is that we are required to make decisions in circumstances that impose time limits using a fraction of the information required to avoid errors. This is critical. We make decisions over time and in contexts in which we observe the client, receive information reported to us by the client and others, and in which we have suspicions or make inferences. We are never playing with a full deck, and there is the added problem that we believe we are.

In order to appreciate the level of uncertainty that is inherent to our views of mental disorders and their management, think about the historical evolution of our theories and conclusions. Reviewing the past 150 years, we are confronted by a number of theories and *facts* that were subsequently shown to be wrong or at least not as definitive as we believed. Here again is evidence for the certainty bias getting us into trouble (e.g., lobotomy, insulin shock, refrigerator mothers, and the safety of benzodiazepines). Our tendency is toward conviction in our views despite historical and other evidence telling us our certainty about anything is susceptible to error at best and dangerous at worst.

We can move so quickly from fact to fiction. For example, the paper by Prasad and colleagues titled "A Decade of Reversal: An Analysis of 146 Contradicted Medical Practices" shows that many treatments that were once taken as dogma have since been discredited by new or more complete information.[24]

The importance of time as a factor intertwined with uncertainty is inescapable yet also rarely recognized. Mental disorders are particularly subject to the effects of time given that they tend to span years and their presentations vary according to phase of illness. This prominence of changing phenomena is easy to miss or underestimate because we often have a fragmented and incomplete view of patients. This is either because we see them briefly in artificial environments or because it is difficult for us to hold a retrospective or prospective view of what may be unfolding before us. As humans, we are better at recognizing change that emerges over short periods, such as hours and days, rather than weeks, months, and years.

A good view of the changing picture over time is provided by the cradle-to-grave health records maintained by family physicians. Individual patients with mental disorders frequently have charts that reveal a multitude of diagnoses from various providers—for example, depression, anxiety, bipolar affective disorder, a personality disorder, fibromyalgia, and post-traumatic stress disorder. This likely reflects the ambiguity of symptoms and their overlap across multiple diagnoses, the fluctuating nature of mental disorders, unrecognized comorbidity, and the impact of these on diagnostic accuracy.

Considering clinical uncertainty constrained by time, we have found the concept of *irreducible uncertainty* delineated by Kenneth Hammond to be extremely useful.[25] Hammond uses irreducible uncertainty to refer to "uncertainty that cannot be reduced by any activity at the moment action is required" (p. 13). Based on this and other definitions, we suggest the following definition in the context of clinical decision making:

> Irreducible uncertainty is the gap between all the information, knowledge, and information processing capacity that the clinician has at the moment they make a judgment or decision and what would be required to make a judgment or decision that is entirely free of error.

Note that the proposed definition ignores the contribution of random error to irreducible uncertainty. This is primarily because our gaps in information and knowledge related to mental health are so cavernous that random error becomes insignificant.

Irreducible uncertainty is a term also used in reference to the variability within population or group-based observations. This is sometimes referred to as statistical uncertainty. It essentially refers to the uncertainty that arises when clinicians attempt to apply group-based data to individual clients. Beyond choosing studies that select subjects that completely reflect an individual's characteristics, this source of uncertainty is irreducible at the moment of the decision and remains irreducible as long as the study informs clinical care. In addition, the gap between the current state of collective knowledge about any subject and a perfect state of understanding it is known as epistemic uncertainty.

When reading the phrase in the proposed definition, "to make a judgment or decision that is entirely free of error," you may have been struck by how unusual it would be to assert, in a clinical domain, that the probability of error in your judgment and decision is zero. If we can bravely admit how frequently we feel certain and think we "know," the ubiquity and power of the certainty bias begin to emerge. Even now, you may be having thoughts such as "I have never considered my judgments to be error free, I just don't think the errors are significant in frequency and impact" or "There is nothing I can do about it anyway. So long as I meet the standard of practice, I am doing the best I can." Welcome to the certainty bias and avoidance of anxiety, respectively!

There are many narratives for why we are so pulled toward definitive answers. Robert Burton, a neurologist, summarizes this predilection as follows: "At bottom, we are pattern recognizers who seek escape from ambiguity and indecision. If a major brain function is to maintain mental homeostasis, it is understandable how stances of certainty can counteract anxiety and apprehension."[1] In addition, he theorizes that certainty triggers the same pleasure and reward centers in the brain as any craving when satisfied. He says that the sensorial signals, emotions, or thoughts that tell us we are on a path to certainty are "qualitatively as powerful as those involved in sex and gambling. One need only look at the self-satisfied smugness of a 'know it all' to suspect that the feeling of certainty can approach the power of addiction." As certainty is rewarding, so uncertainty is distressing. Arie Kruglanski, a social psychologist, defined the need for clear-cut answers and our "aversion toward ambiguity" as a drive toward *cognitive closure*.[4,5,20] We could posit that this drive derives from our ancestors' anxious brains that needed to know when certainty was around the corner to bring some ease but also required anxiety to help keep them alert and alive when it was not. We, the authors, admit an attraction to the coherence of this narrative. At the same time, we are aware that this drive toward explaining the unknown is a compulsion; even while writing a book about uncertainty.

So, where are we? To review, we have the concept of irreducible uncertainty and its application to ourselves as clinicians, and we have the clinical imperative of making decisions at a moment in time when the information necessary to eliminate error is always unavailable. At the same time, we have the incompatible certainty bias and clinician overconfidence.

Given that uncertainty and risk are tightly bound, it is essential to recognize our need for certainty as a bias that largely operates outside of awareness and impairs our ability to perceive gaps in our knowledge.[2] Confronted by ambiguity and, more generally, the need to provide an opinion or decision despite incomplete information, clinicians demonstrate a variety of behaviors. The responses to uncertainty include ignoring the ambiguity, ignoring differential diagnoses, or relying on cross-sectional investigations independent of their applicability.[2,26,27] The consequence of unwarranted certainty is unrecognized error and the failure to learn from practice.

If we agree that without awareness of our certainty bias and its effects our options for decision making and management are narrowed, then perhaps one way to begin working with this is to increase our capacity for both tolerating and recognizing uncertainty. One way to do this is by getting to know our personal signatures that show up when unwarranted certainty is rearing its head or anxiety is arising because we are feeling uncertain. By investigating the common thoughts, emotions, physical sensations, and behaviors that arise, we may be able to take a step back from our tendency to believe everything we think and begin to ask ourselves, "Do we really know what is going on?" or "Are we making assumptions in need of clarification?" or "Are we jumping to conclusions and can we re-frame these as hypotheses?" We can begin to investigate our cognitive style and find out if we are a "fox" (more cautious around decision making and more aware of being error prone) or a "hedgehog" (more optimistic and defensive of our predictions and decision making).[28] Can we get curious about how we meet and relate to uncertainty in clinical practice? This is the bringing of mindful attention to experience.

Unfortunately, attempts at improved awareness and insight are insufficient. If we hope to achieve meaningful shifts in practice, we need something clearer and concrete. We believe it is necessary to enhance the extent to which our field prioritizes risk as a focus for attention in clinical care if we are to reduce mortality and disability stemming from mental disorders.[29,30] Without appreciating the uncertainty inherent to clinical practice and historical failure to reducing harm associated with mental disorders, we can be lulled into superficial risk assessments and unchecked judgments of safety. We may miss the possibility of averting harm to those who are directly under our care and sadly to others. Indeed, the literature on our effectiveness at accurately assessing risk suggests our current approaches require urgent improvement.[31-34]

Therefore, we need to value the acknowledgment of when we don't know, in the interests of our clients. We are not suggesting that we should not act until we are certain. Rather, it is important to act with uncertainty in mind, recognizing that our judgment and decisions are prone to error. These should be continuously scrutinized with a view to reducing the probability of errors that may lead to mortality and morbidity. To that end, by prioritizing the probability of risk, along with related functional impairment and symptoms, we can focus on acute and concrete concerns. The aim is to ensure that we halt the flow of harm to our client while in search of a diagnosis or meeting longer term treatment goals.

We must also explore the contribution of complexity to the uncertainty we continuously face in clinical practice. It is to this complexity that we now turn.

References

1. Lehrer J, Burton R. The certainty bias: A potentially dangerous mental flaw. *Sci Am*. October 9, 2008. https://www.scientificamerican.com/article/the-certainty-bias/#:~:text=The%20 Certainty%20Bias:%20A%20Potentially%20Dangerous%20Mental%20Flaw,sound%20 too%20sure%20of%20themselves.%20October%209,%202008.
2. Burton RA. *On Being Certain: Believing You Are Right Even When You're Not*. New York: St. Martin's Press; 2008.
3. Fernbach PM, Darlow A, Sloman SA. Asymmetries in predictive and diagnostic reasoning. *J Exp Psychol Gen*. 2011;140(2):168–185.
4. Kruglanski AW, Webster DM. Motivated closing of the mind: "Seizing" and "freezing." *Psychol Rev*. 1996;103(2):263–283.
5. Kruglanski AW, Orehek E. The need for certainty as a psychological nexus for individuals and society. In: Hogg MA, Blaylock DL, eds. *Extremism and the Psychology of Uncertainty*. Malden, MA: Wiley-Blackwell; 2012:3–18.
6. Crumlish N, Kelly B. How psychiatrists think. *Adv Psychiatr Treat*. 2009;15:72–79.
7. Saposnik G, Sempere AP, Raptis R, Prefasi D, Selchen D, Maurino J. Decision making under uncertainty, therapeutic inertia, and physicians' risk preferences in the management of multiple sclerosis (DIScUTIR MS). *BMC Neurol*. 2016;16:58.
8. Lau DC. Therapeutic inertia and nihilism. *Can J Diabetes*. 2014;38(5):290–291.
9. Phillips LS, Branch WT, Cook CB, et al. Clinical inertia. *Ann Intern Med*. 2001;135(9):825–834.
10. Khunti K, Gomes MB, Pocock S, et al. Therapeutic inertia in the treatment of hyperglycaemia in patients with type 2 diabetes: A systematic review. *Diabetes Obes Metab*. 2018;20(2):427–437.
11. Lazaro P, Murga N, Aguilar D, Hernandez-Presa MA; INERTIA Study Investigators. Therapeutic inertia in the outpatient management of dyslipidemia in patients with ischemic heart disease: The inertia study. *Rev Esp Cardiol*. 2010;63(12):1428–1437.
12. Mahabaleshwarkar R, Gohs F, Mulder H, et al. Patient and provider factors affecting clinical inertia in patients with type 2 diabetes on metformin monotherapy. *Clin Ther*. 2017;39(8):1658–1670.e6.
13. Man FY, Chen CX, Lau YY, Chan K. Therapeutic inertia in the management of hyperlipidaemia in type 2 diabetic patients: A cross-sectional study in the primary care setting. *Hong Kong Med J*. 2016;22(4):356–364.
14. Rea F, Corrao G, Merlino L, Mancia G. Initial antihypertensive treatment strategies and therapeutic inertia. *Hypertension*. 2018;72(4):846–853.
15. Simon D. Therapeutic inertia in type 2 diabetes: Insights from the PANORAMA study in France. *Diabetes Metab*. 2012;38(Suppl 3):S47–S52.
16. Insel TR. The NIMH Research Domain Criteria (RDoC) Project: Precision medicine for psychiatry. *Am J Psychiatry*. 2014;171(4):395–397.
17. Kendler KS, Zachar P, Craver C. What kinds of things are psychiatric disorders? *Psychol Med*. 2011;41(6):1143–1150.
18. Paris J. *The Intelligent Clinician's Guide to the DSM 5*. New York: Oxford University Press; 2015.

19. Saposnik G. Applying behavioral economics and neuroeconomics to medical education and clinical care. *Can J Neurol Sci*. 2019;46(1):35–37.
20. Webster DM, Kruglanski AW. Cognitive and social consequences of the need for cognitive closure. *Eur Rev Social Psychol*. 1997;8(1):133–173.
21. West AF, West RR. Clinical decision-making: Coping with uncertainty. *Postgrad Med J*. 2002;78(920):319–321.
22. MeSH Browser (2011 MeSH) [Internet]. *Medical subject headings section* [1999; updated August 28, 2010; cited July 8, 2011]. Bethesda, MD: National Library of Medicine. http://www.nlm.nih.gov/mesh/MBrowser.html.
23. Han P, Klein W, Arora N. Varieties of uncertainty in health care: A conceptual taxonomy. *Med Decis Making*. 2011;31(6):828–838.
24. Prasad V, Vandross A, Toomey C, et al. A decade of reversal: An analysis of 146 contradicted medical practices. *Mayo Clin Proc*. 2013;88(8):790–798.
25. Hammond KR. *Human Judgment and Social Policy: Irreducible Uncertainty, Inevitable Error, Unavoidable Injustice*. Kindle ed. New York: Oxford University Press; 1996.
26. Howman M, Walters K, Rosenthal J, Ajjawi R, Buszewicz M. "You kind of want to fix it don't you?" Exploring general practice trainees' experiences of managing patients with medically unexplained symptoms. *BMC Med Educ*. 2016;16:27.
27. Hamer HP, McCallin AM. Cardiac pain or panic disorder? Managing uncertainty in the emergency department. *Nurs Health Sci*. 2006;8(4):224–230.
28. Tetlock PE. *Expert Political Judgment: How Good Is It? How Can We Know?* 2nd ed. Princeton, NJ: Princeton University Press; 2017.
29. Walker ER, McGee RE, Druss BG. Mortality in mental disorders and global disease burden implications: A systematic review and meta-analysis. *JAMA Psychiatry*. 2015;72(4):334–341.
30. Schanda H, Knecht G, Schreinzer D, Stompe T, Ortwein-Swoboda G, Waldhoer T. Homicide and major mental disorders: A 25-year study. *Acta Psychiatr Scand*. 2004;110(2):98–107.
31. Bolton JM, Gunnell D, Turecki G. Suicide risk assessment and intervention in people with mental illness. *BMJ*. 2015;351:h4978. http://www.bmj.com/content/351/bmj.h4978. abstract.
32. Feldman MD, Franks P, Duberstein PR, Vannoy S, Epstein R, Kravitz RL. Let's not talk about it: Suicide inquiry in primary care. *Ann Fam Med*. 2007;5(5):412–418.
33. HIROC. *On-premises suicides/attempts*. Risk Reference Sheet Mental Health. Toronto: HIROC; 2016.
34. Luoma JB, Martin CE, Pearson JL. Contact with mental health and primary care providers before suicide: A review of the evidence. *Am J Psychiatry*. 2002;159(6):909–916.

2

The Brain as a Complex Adaptive System

Perhaps it was something like this that the twentieth century satirist H. L. Mencken was thinking about when he wrote, "For every complex problem there is an answer that is clear, simple, and wrong."

—Delaplane[1]

Complexity limits the accuracy of establishing causation, pattern recognition, and predictions, all three of which are fundamental to clinical practice and the research that informs it. Our minds are so effective at creating the illusion of simplicity that complexity has been universally minimized in the field of mental health. Our aim in this chapter is to introduce complexity and its contribution to objective uncertainty in our domain. We also hope clinicians will gain appreciation for the complexity inherent to mental health care and reduce their vulnerability to confusing this with their own limitations.

Complexity comes in different forms. One of the these is complex adaptive systems (CASs), of which the brain is an archetype. Such systems involve a cacophony of interacting elements that are continuously inducing change. This occurs in both the elements individually and the *system* of elements as a whole. An introductory view of the brain and mind through this lens helps us appreciate the irreducibility of some sources of clinical uncertainty and why complexity is a pragmatic issue in mental health. Very broadly, a CAS is characterized by multiple interdependent and interacting parts, in which even a perfect understanding of the individual parts and their interactions is inadequate to understanding how the system behaves as a unified whole. Practically, this means that when dealing with such entities, what is knowable and predictable about the system and its emergent properties has impenetrable limits.

Using a CAS model to view disruptions to mental health has the added benefit of addressing the brain versus mind conundrum. From a CASs perspective, the mind can be conceptualized as an emergent property of the brain. This unifies divisive arguments while providing a framework that explains why the mind and its disruptions cannot be understood by simply understanding the brain's individual parts and their interactions. A perfect understanding of the brain remains elusive, but even when achieved, it will be insufficient to allow accurate comprehension and prediction of the mind. This suggests greater, not less, skepticism of our theories of mind and its disruptions. In summary, a CAS model would suggest that the brain is not the mind and the mind is not the brain, but it is difficult to have one without the other.

We now discuss some of the properties of CASs and their relationship to the brain and mind. For more complete discussions of these properties, we refer readers to works by other authors.[2,3] For our purposes, we focus on the properties most likely to preclude accurate understanding of the antecedents to disordered mental phenomena and the inability to predict how such phenomena will change, with or without our interventions. These relevant properties are the following:

- Emergence
- Multiple interacting components
- Nonlinearity and unpredictability
- Contagion
- Modularity

Emergence

We have referred periodically to the mind as an emergent property of the brain without an explanation of what this means or how a CAS model supports this view. Emergence can be thought of as the overt manifestation of the interactions between the components of a complex system as a whole—for instance, the music created by an improvisational jazz band. In mental health care, emergence is reflected in the phenotypic manifestation of the disorders we encounter. As mental health clinicians, although we may consider structural or otherwise concrete neuroanatomical aspects of the brain, we are primarily engaged with phenomena of mind. As such, it is important to understand the concept of emergence as it relates to the phenomena we associate with mental disorders.

So, what is emergence? To start, emergence can be understood as "the whole is greater than the sum of its parts," and you would never predict the whole by simply studying the parts. It can be conceived of as a process whereby larger entities and patterns arise through interactions among smaller or simpler entities that themselves do not exhibit the property that ultimately manifests. Emergence is what happens when synergistic effects are not only quantitatively different but also interact to be "qualitatively" different than the combination of the elements in the original system. None of the elements, when taken in isolation, have the qualities of the emergent phenomena. Furthermore, the interactions between elements and the phenomena that emerges are not orchestrated or centrally controlled by any of the elements. For instance, a collection of bees interacting with one another and their environment to build a beehive do so in the absence of any leadership, including the queen bee because she does not direct its construction (or any bee-*haviors*, contrary to popular belief). This is often referred to as spontaneous organization.

One of the most common examples used to illustrate emergence is the phenomena of consciousness. Consciousness arises from the interacting elements of the brain but is not evident in the brain's component parts. Other examples include the changing patterns arising from a flock of starlings in flight or the property of wetness when a sufficient number of water molecules interact under the right conditions. To further illustrate the distinction between quantitative and qualitative difference, consider that the mass of a cup of water is a simple addition of the mass of each molecule. It is easy to predict the collective mass of the cup of water by knowing the mass of a water molecule. What is not predicted is the property of wetness. Incidentally, the hardness of ice is also not predicted by its constituent parts.

Returning to the property of spontaneous organization or reorganization, one of the interesting aspects of it is that some perturbations or interactions from within or without the CAS can result in a new emergent state that is prolonged. Applying this to the brain and mind, we can consider that some spontaneous organization in response to events inside or outside the brain could lead to a change in the emergent pattern of the mind, such as symptoms of mental disorders. This would certainly be consistent with the difficulty we are having in finding biological correlates to the majority of mental disorders.

A concerning aspect to spontaneous organization is that it is possible that the longer the system retains its spontaneously organized pattern, the more difficult it may be to alter it to a more functional state. It is easy to see how this relates to early intervention in mental illness and its importance.

Remember that it is not only those whom we identify as sick who may reflect this loss of malleability. We may all exhibit a degree of this kind of rigidity in our beliefs, reactions, and behaviors. However, the extent to which this occurs in those with mental disorders conveys suffering, impairment, and dysfunction that usually go beyond variations in cultural values and beliefs.

Multiple Interacting Components

> With its billions of interconnected neurons, whose interactions change from millisecond to millisecond, the human brain is an archetypal complex system.
>
> —Miguel Nicolelis[4]

If we think about the brain's component parts and their number, what we are confronted with is staggering. Counting neurons exclusively and ignoring all the other cells that compose the brain's network, we are still left with a gross estimate of more than 86 billion neurons. These interact through an estimated 1 trillion connections. A trillion connections are a million, million connections—a number so large our brains are unable to understand what this means. So, let's try to put a trillion connections into perspective by translating the numbers into events and time. If we were to send an infinitesimally small robot to weave its way through each and every connection within the brain, at a speed of 1 million connections per day, it would take this industrious little robot approximately 2,740 years to complete its journey. Conceiving of this web of connections as effectively infinite lays the foundation for a discussion of an important property of CASs—that of nonlinearity and the difficulty in predicting what a system such as this will do or explaining what it has done.

Nonlinearity and Unpredictability

Nonlinearity means that a complex system does not predictably respond the same way to the same stimulus at different moments in time. It plays a major role in the difficulty of accurately explaining why or how a complex system came to be in its current state or to predict the system's future behavior. This unpredictability is one of the most important properties for clinicians to appreciate. As a result, it is very difficult to say what the state of the system might be in the future, what it might have been in the past, and even understand the immediate state before us. This means that our search for coherence and causal explanations for our current observations of the system are prone to error.

Major contributors to nonlinearity are the continuous changes within the system's components, their connections, and the ubiquity of feedback loops between interacting elements.

Feedback Loops

A system, as discussed previously, can be described as complex when it contains multiple components or elements that are interconnected and interacting. Such systems are complicated (with many parts) and complex (nonlinear), unlike, for example, the Krebs cycle, which, although complicated, is linear and predictable. This is not the case with the feedback loops in CASs that, although they may amplify or inhibit, can also change the quality of the signal and its repercussions. A simplistic and gross example is the observation that human beings can interpret physiological arousal as either fear or excitement depending on the context, expectations, interpretation, or other factors. These elements influence each other's functioning or behavior in a multitude of perpetual *feedback loops.* The combination of components and their reverberating interactions create a system that is in a continual state of change. Changes in complex systems are especially substantial in response to internal or external stimulation of the system. When the complex system is malleable and responds to stimuli with the development of a new pattern (spontaneous organization), it can be classified as a CAS.

These feedback loops within the brain occur at multiple levels of granularity. Neurons constantly change and act differently depending on inputs at any given moment. These continuously shifting components, and the adaptation to ongoing stimuli combined, result in the nonlinear dynamics of the brain. This is all to say that using a few static variables [e.g., *Diagnostic and Statistical Manual of Mental Disorders* (DSM) criteria or formulations] is a simplistic attempt to describe or explain emergent mental phenomena.

Change and adaptation in the brain also occur over varying durations. For instance, think of the inhibition or stimulation of neuronal firing that happens over milliseconds. Then contrast this to the underlying neural substrates that give rise to varying emotions over minutes and hours in response to experiences. Last, consider the development of a clinician's knowledge, skills, and expertise in professional practice that occurs over years. If we think we fully grasp the complexity of the brain and can successfully understand the emergent mind it gives rise to—we are probably wrong.

Clinical Implications

So, how might the property of nonlinearity relate to mental disorders and their management? There are many ways, but a clinical example may be useful. Wittenborn et al. discuss the complexity of unipolar depression and the feedback mechanisms that underlie and contribute to its persistence.[5] Through an examination of the literature, they found that 93% of more than 12,000 articles examined only one variable, each related to causation of the disease, reflecting a "common cause" model and linear view of the etiology of depression. We can see this as an attempt to develop a parsimonious view of a disorder. However, the nonlinearity and other properties of CASs tend to defy simplification. Once we expose the person and their brain to their environment, we increase the levels of complexity by adding additional CASs into the mix, all interacting and influencing each other in an unpredictable manner. So why is this of relevance? A linear, reductionist view of a clinical presentation that does not take into account the degree of complexity of the brain and other CASs with which it interacts cannot expect to inform adequate assessment or treatment. Nor can it provide a complete and accurate causal explanation. More recently, there appears to be a move away from simple causation models of disorders, such as depression, toward others that consider "complex causal mechanisms that underlie psychiatric syndromes."[6,7]

We might be lulled by our certainty bias to imagine that our current knowledge of the brain and other complex systems is sufficient to decipher how these multiple systems (e.g., biological, environmental, and social) interact to give rise to both healthy and pathological states of mind. Such a belief is premature. We haven't even figured out how the brain gives rise to the mind, much less how the environment influences the development of changes in the brain. Clinically, however, we often function as if we do.

For example, one of the most common skills that is expected of mental health clinicians is to know how to work with an explanatory model that is touted as providing an inclusive causal formulation for a person's clinical presentation. Engel's biopsychosocial model is asserted as necessary to effectively understand *why* a person is presenting the way they are. This model presumes the human being can be understood using a few variables that consist of unverified content and causal connections. This assertion is inconsistent with the nonlinearity and lack of predictability of complex systems. Training, however, supports the belief that clinicians can have enough confidence in their formulation to base all future treatment plans on it.

The ease with which we underestimate the irreducible uncertainty that CASs introduce into our clinical explanatory models is ironically demonstrated by

Wittenborn and coauthors.[5] They discuss the potential effect and interaction of feedback loops between complex systems in depression. They use the example of a putative relationship between economic difficulties and depression as an illness. The authors refer to two factors as *causing* the illness of depression: "two causal links create a reinforcing loop which may trap an individual in increasing financial hardship and depression" (p. 4).[5] These authors, attentive to the limitations of a linear, reductionist approach to managing mental disorders, nonetheless reveal how deeply ingrained is our human tendency toward linear thinking.

In contrast, we believe CAS theory would suggest that numerous factors would potentially be associated with both emerging phenomena (in this case, in the depressed person) and any stimulus (intervention or otherwise). This would then result in unpredictable changes to the phenomena of interest. There is likely to be complex heterogeneity in antecedents to depressive illness in the individual as well as in the responses to interventions across individuals. Indeed, this is consistent with the variability we experience in working with people in clinical practice. This inherent nonlinearity may be one of the reasons why people with ostensibly the same illness may experience very different signs, symptoms, risks, and altered functioning. When we invoke the concept of *the same illness*, we must recognize the number of assumptions that go into our existing diagnostic systems. We discuss this in-depth in Chapter 4. As clinicians, if we were able to fully appreciate the nonlinear dynamic nature of the complex systems underlying the disorders we are managing, this might reduce our tendency toward simplistic conclusions and unwarranted certainty in our impressions.

Implications for Clinical Uncertainty

Where and under what circumstances does uncertainty arise in the management of mental health and addictions viewed through the lens of CASs? We must remember the properties of multiple interacting components, nonlinearity, feedback loops, and their dynamic nature. From this perspective, we can begin to understand what it means to work with a person who presents in an undifferentiated manner, ostensibly with a mental disorder. It means we must consider many variables at once, and these include but are not confined to issues that revolve around the patient such as duration and severity of symptoms; the past if relevant; and the patient's age, sex, gender, level of education, medical conditions, other comorbidities, substance dependence, and cognitive impairments.[8] There are also issues to consider that relate to social interactions, such as the effect of mental illness on relationships (e.g., inter-personal difficulties and conflict), language and cultural differences, current context (e.g., availability of supports), or an inability to care for dependents. Last, interactions with the health care system, such as "experiential challenges including difficulty navigating services and the need for a care manager, lack of access to providers, heavy utilization of services, and higher healthcare costs" (p. 2),[8] are also aspects of clinical complexity.

We must consider all of this and more in our judgments of risk and ability to function, and then make decisions about management. This then introduces other variables, such as medication(s), admission to hospital, demands of third-party payers, and the risk of a complaint or a lawsuit, that will further evoke change in this complex human system. No wonder most health care providers are averse to the management of mental disorders.[9]

Although the research examining depression and other psychiatric conditions as CASs is early, given our failure to consistently reduce their public health impact, a strong case can be made for ongoing investigation into alternate approaches to mood and other mental disorders. We will propose an approach or schema to help clinicians organize their thinking and manage the complexity of their patients or clients, particularly when at risk. But first, let's continue our exploration of nonlinearity and unpredictability followed by discussion of other aspects of CASs and their relevance to mental health care.

Nonlinearity is a particularly important property of complexity. This relates to the interplay of the innumerable variables that result in the inability to accurately ascertain causation and treatment response in a clinical sphere. When working with CASs, we are limited to discussing probabilities rather than determinable events. Clinicians consider diagnoses to be conclusions based on their synthesis of available information. However, a retrospective review of diagnoses in an unfolding mental disorder frequently reveals a changing landscape of conclusions over time. For example, an adolescent may present with what initially appears to be an anxiety disorder (based on specific phenomena), only to present with manic symptoms and delusions (suggested by other phenomena) a few years later, resulting in another set of diagnostic possibilities.

A linear and retrospective perspective in such instances may invoke the diagnostic conclusion of a comorbid anxiety and bipolar affective disorder. It might also be asserted that the clinician failed to obtain all available information in the first place. In other words, the implication is that one or more discrete diagnoses accurately denote the system, and if we simply made no errors in collecting all the data, we would be able to establish the correct diagnosis going forward. In contrast, viewing the story via a CAS model, we would anticipate that our conclusions are likely to be wrong at any given moment, that all we can fairly state is a series of probabilities, and that the perpetually dynamic nature of the system suggests that the person's presentation will change.

When we perceive that a patient's presentation is qualitatively different from one point in time to another, we may blame ourselves for missing something (which may be true), but often we have simply not accounted for the nonlinearity and lack of predictability of the systems with which we are working. If nothing else, nonlinearity can remind us not to confuse our narratives and beliefs with truth.

And yet, humans are somewhat predictable for periods of time, whether they are sick or well. This can be deceiving for clinicians and encourage our tendency toward certainty. We forget that the probability of multiple events over time does not necessarily translate into the predictability of discrete events at any given moment for any given person.

We are, in reality, like meteorologists wrestling to extract reliable predictions from complex weather systems. What might we clinicians learn from them? The probability of error in weather prediction is manageable for approximately 2–5 days into the future, beyond which the probability of predictive error skyrockets. Although those with mental disorders may not be as unpredictable as the weather, it reminds us that the certainty we approach them with is clearly unwarranted. Having said this, the National Weather Service (NWS) in the United States has only recently been able to achieve this degree of accuracy through the evolution of computer modeling. The computer models in turn require enormous numbers of observations with which to work. According to the NWS, it takes in 192,000 observations from surface stations, 2,700 from ships, 18,000 from weather buoys, 115,000 from aircraft, 250,000 from balloons, and 140 million from satellites.[10] This doesn't include information incorporated from other international networks. The data are then updated (remember weather and climate are CASs and therefore always changing) at least *every hour*. Compared to meteorologists, the relatively meager data available to clinicians about the individual and the disorders they are faced with is sadly lacking. Evan Collins quipped, "This begs the question, is the DSM akin to computer modeling or The Farmer's Almanac" (E. Collins, personal communication, July 6, 2019). Contagion and modularity are two other properties of CASs that help understand the uncertainty faced by clinicians. Contagion refers to a process by which phenomena within a CAS can spread very quickly. This occurs because the system's components or elements are tightly connected, and the phenomena can propagate rapidly, spreading to involve an entire system.

To illustrate the relevance of this, imagine someone who begins to manifest disordered connections in their thinking. This thinking may progress to a fixed, well-organized paranoid delusion, subsequently affecting the person's emotions, behaviors, and interactions. Over time, other people may be incorporated into the delusion. This could be construed as contagion and conceivably reflect spread of a process in the neural networks of the brain.

In contrast, the property of modularity is one reason why phenomena do not always spread to the whole system. Modularity speaks to the fact that although such a system is well connected, there are subsets of elements within it that are more connected to each other than to the remainder of the system. Consider the example of intraconnections of the cerebellum and the intraconnections of Broca's area related to speech. A disruption of Broca's area does not necessarily influence the cerebellum or vice versa, despite the global connectedness within the brain.

Consider a less concrete clinical illustration involving phenomena of the mind that currently have no observable neural correlates. Delusional parasitosis is a syndrome wherein an individual has a fixed belief that they are infected with parasites despite no physical evidence of this. This belief may be extremely specific to the parasite itself—for instance, larva, mold spore inhalation, or bedbugs. A relatively *modular* disorder, it is usually narrow, well demarcated, and frequently monosymptomatic. To further illustrate, a person presented to one of the authors with this disorder with unsupported beliefs and disabling worry about bedbugs. When traveling, the person expressed no concern about swimming in foreign waters or lying on the beach (both places one might be worried about parasites other than bedbugs). This circumscribed pattern of symptoms could be conceived of as modularity within the emergent mind and, by implication, indicative of modularity within the brain. This does not mean that one day we will find circumscribed neural areas or connections that are specialized in reality testing nascent fears of bedbug infestations. Despite modularity, emergent phenomena, by definition, are difficult to localize to discrete areas within a CAS.

Instead, contagion and modularity relate to differing levels of connectedness between components of the system. This is regardless of location, although the most probable connections are those that are most proximal. Furthermore, not all perturbations or stimuli will have a lasting effect on the system's behavior. The creation of a new pattern (e.g., the development of the delusional parasitosis at the level of mind) requires a system to reorganize spontaneously. Spontaneous reorganization is characterized by the emergence of a new pattern in the absence of any central control. Broadly speaking, all that is required is a stimulus of some kind. Spontaneous reorganization refers to this new observable pattern. Understanding the concepts of contagion, modularity, and spontaneous reorganization may assist in making sense of the variation within and across mental disorders.

The interdependence of CASs means that in clinical practice our thinking needs to be perpetually provisional. When working with our patients, we should remember that neither they nor their symptoms are static. Complexity suggests that clinical causal formulations are either wrong or incomplete, and no amount of information about the patient's history will change the fallibility. In Chapter 3, we expand on the potential relevance of complexity to clinical practice.

References

1. Delaplane KS. Emergent properties in the honey bee superorganism. *Bee World*. 2017;94(1):8–15.
2. Mitchell M. *Complexity: A Guided Tour*. Oxford University Press; 2011.
3. Morowitz H. *The Mind, The Brain And Complex Adaptive Systems*. First ed. Taylor and Francis Group; 1994.
4. BrainyQuote. Miguel Nicolelis quotes. https://www.brainyquote.com/authors/miguel-nicolelis-quotes. 2021.
5. Wittenborn AK, Rahmandad H, Rick J, Hosseinichimeh N. Depression as a systemic syndrome: mapping the feedback loops of major depressive disorder. *Psychol Med*. 2016;46(3):551–562.
6. Insel TR. The NIMH Research Domain Criteria (RDoC) Project: Precision medicine for psychiatry. *Am J Psychiatry*. 2014;171(4):395–397.
7. Kendler KS, Zachar P, Craver C. What kinds of things are psychiatric disorders? *Psychol Med*. 2011;41(6):1143–1150.
8. Schaink AK, Kuluski K, Lyons RF, et al. A scoping review and thematic classification of patient complexity: Offering a unifying framework. *J Comorb*. 2012;2:1–9.
9. Brown T, Ryland H. Recruitment to psychiatry: A global problem. *BJPsych Int*. 2019;16(1):1–3.
10. National Weather Service. About the NWS. https://www.weather.gov. Updated 2019. Accessed September 20, 2019.

3

Complexity in Clinical Practice

The way in which we have been considering complexity is daunting and goes far beyond the ways we tend to think about it clinically. For instance, in the research literature, the most common variable considered to connote "patient complexity" is diagnostic comorbidity.[1-5] Addressing patient complexity goes beyond comorbidity and involves many interacting, unpredictable elements that may be subsumed within three major areas: the patient, their interaction with the social system, and the health care system itself. In a scoping review, Schaink and others derived a comprehensive list of variables associated with "patient complexity."[5] This is important because we need to take into account other aspects beyond comorbidities when thinking about treatment decisions. Although comorbidities add to a person's presentation and assessment, we argue that this construct is both incomplete and simplistic when applied to mental disorders and how we might approach them. If we think only in terms of comorbid diagnoses when judging client complexity, then we ignore a whole host of other influences that challenge our ability to assess and manage clients effectively.

The human limitations in data processing mean that we can cognitively manage only a small number of variables at any time. We must also deal with our knowledge gaps and those that are epistemological. These factors create challenges that may contribute to our reductionistic tendencies, our need for certainty, and the necessity to narrowly focus during judgment and decision making.

Respecting our limitations is unlikely to be sufficient for a comprehensive understanding of the emergent properties of the system with which we are concerned. We suggest that in addition to acknowledging that the brain is a complex adaptive system, our clinical processes need to incorporate the inevitability of error in clinical attempts to integrate multiple complex adaptive systems such as the person, their environment, society, and so on. In addition, the people with whom we interact become part of a health care system, influence it, and are influenced by it. These are added levels of complexity that go beyond the disorder.

Are there concrete manifestations that complexity is ignored in everyday clinical practice? We believe there are and that we often don't see them. It is hidden in things we take for granted as fact. These include the immutable nature of diagnostic categories, the tendency to view people's states as fixed, and the view that it is sufficient to focus on a small subset of the phenomena. We often get caught up in the probability that one aspect of a case is true and that one variable has primacy. We forget that our knowledge is incomplete, and it is the *complete* picture we need if we are to improve our chance of asking the right questions and providing meaningful assistance. In the words of C. N. Adichie, "The problem with stereotypes is not that they are untrue but rather they are incomplete. They make one story become the only story."[6] In this light, psychiatric diagnoses may be conceptualized as codified stereotypes we associate with those with mental disorders.

Think for a moment about the term *borderline personality disorder* and the stigmatizing characteristics that come to mind about someone given that diagnosis. Specifically, consider how a health care provider might react to such a person who presents to the emergency department after having cut their arm, requiring stitches. This recalls the public criticism that psychiatry affixes "labels" and the potential stigma these invoke. This may be an expression of frustration with being viewed in a limited and prejudicial way. Although we might argue that we clinicians are unbiased and dispassionately focused on the constellation of signs and symptoms, we know this is untrue. It is difficult for us to consistently achieve a comprehensive picture of a person's health status if our view is narrowed by a priori categories and prejudices. This is the danger of the single story combined with the certainty bias.

Complexity Operationalized

To review, clinical or patient complexity is generally viewed in much simpler terms than suggested by complexity science, and it refers primarily to patient comorbidities, psychosocial factors, and the person's cross-sectional and longitudinal context.[7] It is the expectation that all the interacting factors can be successfully synthesized by a clinician. However, this is grossly at odds with the properties of complex adaptive systems. What clinicians face is much larger than the often-limiting stories we have or categories we use to think about our clients.

Let's consider side effects as a concrete example of what we are actually dealing with. We are all familiar with side effects of any biological, social, or psychological intervention. We manage them on a day-to-day basis and address them to the best of our ability. But side effects can also be conceptualized as nonlinear manifestations of complex adaptive systems. We may not get the results we are seeking and get others we weren't looking for. To appreciate this, we need to deconstruct aspects of the system with which we are interacting. Side effects are *simply* the effects of an intervention we don't want. But they are not simple. For the purpose of discussion, we focus on side effects associated with pharmacological interventions because they are considerably more concrete and overt than side effects related to psychosocial treatments.

To begin, let's enumerate a subset of the variables that is involved in side effects. The first is the human being and whether, how, when, or with what they take the medication prescribed and how all these factors interact—a dynamic system. Interacting with the person is the medication itself and its interaction with multiple components (e.g., the person, concomitant drugs and conditions, the medication itself, taking it, excreting it, etc.), all connected by feedback loops that ultimately give rise to *side effects*. In addition, the system will adapt to the side effects in multiple ways. The person may stop taking the medication because it is unpleasant, or they feel better; the unwanted effects fade or the person responds to the drug in a way that ensures continuation. So, thus far, even with this limited illustration, complexity begins to come into clearer view. It is this nonlinear component of complex systems that challenges our ability to accurately predict outcomes when modifying even one variable within an entire system. It is no wonder that we rely on stories and explanatory models to assist in bringing coherence to our thinking and decision making.

Implications for Judgment and Decision Making

Recognizing that the brain is a complex adaptive system means we should expect that our clinical judgment and decisions are likely to be wrong or incomplete. They thus require continuous scrutiny, review, and testing. In this way, our clinical impressions and plans become works in progress rather than finished products. This fundamental shift may help reduce a myriad of errors in our thinking related to cognitive dispositions to respond (CDRs), such as anchoring, availability bias, and a plethora of others. Rather than keeping in mind the list of CDRs, it might be easier to learn to recognize the constellation of thoughts, emotions, body sensations, and impulses to act that signal we are feeling certain. We might then be more curious about presenting phenomena and more open to accepting information that suggests our conclusions require revision. This shift in view might serve to keep us on our toes, particularly when we are following patients with mental disorders over the long term.

Staying with the elements of complex systems as they relate to mental disorders, we can now begin to translate complexity into decision making. We can imagine that a disruption to mental health arises from unknown stimuli or interactions resulting in nonlinear adaptations that ultimately lead to emergent phenomena. The clinician becomes aware of some of the emergent phenomena, communicated by the patient, usually in a linear manner that lulls them into experiencing an illusion of clarity. Our premise is that a complex adaptive system model of the brain and mind makes it impossible to assert causation of any mental disorder with any certainty. Similarly, the assertion of an accurate diagnosis in mental health is severely constrained by complexity. In contrast, usual clinical practice is to attempt to formulate the person and their presentation in a variety of ways. Clinicians believe that understanding the origins and why the person before them is sick will definitively guide treatment.

The most ubiquitous approach to formulation and decision making, as mentioned previously, is Engel's biopsychosocial model.[8] This is a narrative causal model, commonly used in psychiatry but which has several critics. Of interest, Lehman et al. have proposed a rethinking of the model that explicitly takes into account that, in medicine, it is important to bring attention to the patient as a complex and dynamic entity exposed to many interacting variables intra- and interpersonally.[9,10]

The *Diagnostic and Statistical Manual of Mental Disorders* (DSM) is also commonly used as if it were an explanation for a disordered mind and its manifestations, when it is simply a system of classification.[11] For example, we assess someone with a collection of symptoms and find they fit under the diagnosis of major depressive disorder. We then may believe we now know what they have, why they are behaving the way they are (e.g., social withdrawal or poor hygiene), and how the person will behave in the future. We become satisfied that the picture of the condition is complete, precluding further exploration. It is more accurate to say that we have collected only a small number of emergent phenomena to which we have quickly affixed a label.

Phenomena that we have organized into a nosology for ease of discussion and research have evolved into *truths* or facts that we take for granted as immutable when they are neither necessarily true nor immutable. Although both the biopsychosocial model and DSM are attempts to help us formulate and think about our patients, they can result in narrowed, sloppy thinking and foster unwarranted certainty.

Summary

In this chapter, we introduced the concept of complex adaptive systems using the brain and mind to illustrate key properties. We discussed the properties of complex systems that may be particularly relevant to mental disorders, their assessment, and their treatment. We used simple clinical examples to illustrate the relevance. We underscored how even a little understanding of complex systems helps appreciate the degree of objective uncertainty in mental health care. Last, we briefly discussed two common ways in which clinicians formulate their impressions and introduced some limitations of these resulting from the degree of complexity and uncertainty in mental health.

In Chapter 4, we turn our attention to the problem of prioritizing diagnosis in clinical practice.

References

1. Deruaz-Luyet A, N'Goran AA, Tandjung R, et al. Multimorbidity in primary care: Protocol of a national cross-sectional study in Switzerland. *BMJ Open*. 2015;5(10):e009165.
2. Hughes LD, McMurdo ME, Guthrie B. Guidelines for people not for diseases: The challenges of applying UK clinical guidelines to people with multimorbidity. *Age Ageing*. 2013;42(1):62–69.
3. Man MS, Chaplin K, Mann C, et al. Improving the management of multimorbidity in general practice: Protocol of a cluster randomised controlled trial (The 3D Study). *BMJ Open*. 2016;6(4):e011261.
4. Manning E, Gagnon M. The complex patient: A concept clarification. *Nurs Health Sci*. 2017;19(1):13–21.
5. Schaink AK, Kuluski K, Lyons RF, et al. A scoping review and thematic classification of patient complexity: Offering a unifying framework. *J Comorb*. 2012;2:1–9.
6. TED (Global) Talk (Producer), & Adichie, C. N. (Director). (2009). *The danger of a single story*. [Video/DVD] Accessed August 2019.
7. Mezzich JE, Salloum IM. Clinical complexity and person-centered integrative diagnosis. *World Psychiatry*. 2008;7(1):1–2.
8. Engel GL. The need for a new medical model: A challenge for biomedicine. *Science*. 1977;196(4286):129–136.
9. Guillemin M, Barnard E. George Libman Engel: The biopsychosocial model and the construction of medical practice. In: Collyer F, ed. *The Palgrave Handbook of Social Theory in Health, Illness and Medicine*. Palgrave Macmillan; 2015:236–250.
10. Lehman BJ, David DM, Gruber JA. Rethinking the biopsychosocial model of health: Understanding health as a dynamic system. *Social Personality Psychol Compass*. 2017;11(8):e12328.
11. Paris J. *The Intelligent Clinician's Guide to the DSM-5*. Oxford University Press; 2015.

4
Limitations of Prioritizing Diagnosis

> The idea of the sacred is quite simply one of the most conservative notions in any culture, because it seeks to turn other ideas—uncertainty, progress, change—into crimes.
>
> —Salman Rushdie

As discussed previously, uncertainty in the management of mental disorders is ubiquitous. Until humans have successfully unraveled the enigma of the brain and mind, our guiding nosologies will continue to bake error into every version. As such, a discussion of uncertainty would be incomplete without exploring the influence of the *Diagnostic and Statistical Manual of Mental Disorders* (DSM) on clinical certitude. In this chapter, we discuss the current classification of mental disorders, its clinical advantages and disadvantages, and its relationship to assessment error.

Discussing nosology within a framework of objective uncertainty is critical because both medicine and clinical psychology are governed by the principle that treatment begins with diagnosis. Consequently, nosology influences every aspect of clinical care, from funding applicable research to making individualized treatment decisions. Numerous factors mediate the degree to which clinicians can depend on a diagnosis to guide their decisions. Some of these factors are embedded as hidden assumptions that increase our vulnerability to unjustified confidence in our diagnoses. The following are a few assumptions underlying the diagnostic axiom that are especially pertinent to managing mental disorders:

- A diagnosis has incontrovertible validity.
- An accurate diagnosis is attainable.
- An accurate diagnosis is verifiable.
- The diagnosis is unambiguous and discrete.
- The diagnosis is not altered by comorbidities.

- The diagnosis is immutable.
- Interventions for the diagnosis target etiology.
- Interventions are specific and discrete to the diagnosis.
- Clinical judgment is accurate.

In addition, there are many mediating factors to making a diagnosis and subsequent treatment decisions. These include, but are not limited to, time, priorities, degree of cognitive bias, subjectivity (the client's and the clinician's), and the unquestioned deference to enigmatic and unaided clinical judgment.

Time, for example, is a significant variable that we as clinicians may not fully appreciate. The harm or impact of important sequelae of a mental health condition may arise long before an accurate diagnosis has been identified. It may be months or years before the upper limit of diagnostic clarity is achieved. Even then, diagnoses are subject to change over the life span, across providers, with different methods of assessment, and depending on the phase of illness. We also know that mental disorders include fluctuating phenomena that clinicians may not receive reports about or observe directly. Invariably, clinicians never have more than a snapshot of their patient's actual condition obtained in a clinical setting.

Aspects of an assessment that clinicians prioritize, often without awareness, may influence outcomes. Theoretically, the clinical priorities are to reduce harm, manage functional impairments, and relieve suffering. Arriving at a diagnosis, however, tends to be the real priority. This is reflected in the fact that clinical research is funded according to diagnosis and that research into diagnostic instruments and methods far exceeds research focused on identifying and/or mitigating risk of harm and disability. In many places, a physician cannot admit a patient to hospital without making and documenting a diagnosis. In contrast, clinicians are not required to determine and document a patient's risk of harm, ability to function, or degree of suffering in order to proceed with that admission. This latter aspect of health care systems is an especially overt demonstration of the extent to which diagnosis is prioritized above all other aspects of assessment. It also illuminates the high level of certainty that diagnoses are the key piece of information the system requires to effectively respond to patient needs. This prioritization may be misguided and have devastating consequences for hospital admissions related to mental disorders because harm and disability are relegated to afterthoughts. Admissions in mental health are exclusively required for the purpose of reducing the risk of harm to self and others. Otherwise, mental disorders can be treated in ambulatory settings. And yet it is diagnosis that is both prioritized and mandatory for an admission to be accepted.

In addition, diagnostic methodologies for assessing mental disorders are susceptible to error and impervious to verification because there are no objective tests independent of human observation and subjective reporting. We do have assessment tools such as inventories, specific assessment questions, full assessments such as the Structured Clinical Interview for DSM (SCID) or the Mini-International Neuropsychiatric Interview, and early use of digital biomarkers correlating with cognitive measures and mood. When these fail to elucidate the diagnosis, reliance remains on clinical judgment as the gold standard. In no other branch of medicine are clinicians faced with this level of ambiguity and inability to verify diagnoses.

We now examine the primary nosology used for diagnosing mental disorders.

The Nosology

Internationally, the World Health Organization (WHO)'s *International Classification of Disease* (ICD) is "the diagnostic classification standard for all clinical and research purposes" and "defines the universe of diseases, disorders, injuries and other related health conditions."[1] WHO began to devote more attention to mental disorders after 1960 and since 1978 has partnered with the United States to improve the classification and diagnosis of mental disorders and alcohol- and drug-related disorders. The evolution of the WHO ICD section on mental disorders and the evolution of the DSM have become closely linked over the decades, with the result that the differences between the ICD-11 released in 2018[2] and the DSM-5 released in 2013[3] are minor. From the perspective of objective uncertainty, neither the ICD-11 nor the DSM-5 can transcend the deficits in our existing knowledge. Consequently, they are equally limited by the absence of validity, vis-à-vis nature, and verifiability of their diagnoses. Here, we mean verifiability beyond consensus at the level of the nosology or clinician agreement. To simplify our discussion, we have chosen to focus on the DSM given its prominence in North America and the authors' familiarity with it.

Most clinicians are familiar with the long-standing controversies surrounding the DSM. The development and release of the DSM-5 revealed that these abound for the scholars and researchers informing the DSM's authors. Disagreements and deep divides have been a part of the DSM since the development of the first clinically applicable version in the form of DSM-III. Our aim in this chapter is to explore the sources of uncertainty embedded within the DSM, how we use it, how we extract the data from the patient, and the fragility of the resulting clinical conclusions. Likewise, this means we must discuss the utility of the DSM, or lack thereof, as it relates to undifferentiated presentations or to those that change over time.

The fact that the DSM is primarily a consensus document is, in itself, a reflection of the irreducible uncertainty in our current understanding of mental disorders. This is not to question the credentials of the manual's many contributors and their thorough approach to collating and debating the diagnoses listed in it. To the contrary, despite the expertise and research that they sifted through for more than a decade, scientists and clinicians could still cogently argue for incompatible conclusions to inform the DSM-5. Given that the DSM's diagnoses are the foundation of clinical care and the research that guides it, this means that mental health practice rests upon the fragile foundation of a crude nosology.

Disagreements become apparent early in the DSM-5. Within its first few pages, the tone changes from the Introduction, which acknowledges the inherent uncertainty in the DSM, to a dogmatic tone in the Use of the Manual. These sections appear to contradict themselves and one another. The initially humble tone of the Introduction expresses that the evolution of the DSM has resulted in the recognition that "a too-rigid categorical system does not capture clinical experience" and that "the boundaries between many disorder 'categories' are more fluid over the life course than DSM-IV recognized, and many symptoms assigned to a single disorder may occur, at varying levels of severity, in many other disorders" (p. 5).[3] In addition, "The simple and linear organization (referring to the DSM itself) that best supports clinical practice may not fully capture the complexity and heterogeneity of mental disorders" (p. 12).[3] Toward the conclusion of the Introduction, the authors discuss changes made to DSM-5 to "enhance diagnostic specificity." This involves the elimination of the *not otherwise specified* (NOS) designation when a disorder does not meet diagnostic criteria, replacing it with options for clinicians to "use: *other specified disorder* and *unspecified disorder*" (p. 15).[3] The former is used when the clinician provides a reason, and the latter is used when the clinician does not. Note that this "differentiation . . . is based on the clinician's decision, providing maximum flexibility for diagnosis" (p. 16).[3]

We find it difficult to understand how it is possible to enhance both diagnostic specificity and flexibility at the same time, particularly when it is based on subjective judgment and flawed assessment methods. Beyond the susceptibility of judgment to numerous biases and error, it defeats the purpose of a nosology to suggest that the final arbiter of a correct diagnosis is the momentary judgment of a clinician. Nonetheless, even when clinicians are explicitly instructed to adhere to criteria, diagnostic agreement between clinicians varies from 0.98 to 0.12 (k coefficients on a scale of 0 to 1).[4] This roughly translates into agreements that range from 12% to 98%. Overall, the degree of clinician diagnostic agreement, at a level of diagnostic specificity commonly used in clinical practice, was found to be 0.57.

Critically, disagreement in diagnosis between clinicians translates into diagnostic error. A disagreement means that at least one clinician has made a wrong diagnosis. It doesn't rule out that both clinicians are wrong—thus representing two diagnostic errors—but it does rule out that both are correct because we can't be half right. According to the National Academies of Sciences, Engineering, and Medicine, a correct diagnosis requires that it be both complete and accurate.[5] This means that, overall, clinicians concluded the wrong diagnosis 43% of the time. The latter is worrisome, but the discordantly high levels of confidence clinicians had in their diagnoses found by Sartorius et al. and other studies is more concerning.[4]

Our premise is that the complexity and objective uncertainty related to managing mental disorders predict a high probability of error despite our best efforts. Consequently, if clinicians fully appreciated the degree of uncertainty within which they function, their level of confidence in their diagnostic judgments and decisions would be very modest. To the contrary, dependent on the disorder, the proportion of physicians who report being "very confident or moderately confident" in their diagnosis ranged from 56.3% to 100%, with the average being 91.1%.[6–10] Based on this literature, deferring to clinician judgment as the final arbiter for the correct diagnosis means that patients will receive a wrong diagnosis 43% of the time by a clinician who has only a 9% chance of appreciating they might be wrong. This level of unwarranted confidence leaves the clinician at risk of premature diagnostic closure, an erroneously narrow differential diagnosis, and failing to consider appropriate treatment options.

The inconsistencies in the introductory sections of the DSM-5 reflect the ambiguity of our diagnoses and the dependence on clinicians' fallible judgments. This raises obvious concerns regarding the manual's reliability but also its validity. Kendell and Jablensky discuss mental disorders as "syndromes" for which diagnostic categories have limited validity vis-à-vis nature but perhaps greater utility, "by virtue of the information about outcome, treatment response and etiology that they convey."[10] In their reference to mental disorders as syndromes, clinicians are reminded that our nosology is not predicated upon etiology and thus diagnoses paired with causal formulations are especially unreliable. However, we tend to quickly lose this view with clinicians and researchers automatically reifying these phenomena as well understood diseases. We suggest that DSM diagnostic categories

unintentionally create the illusion of providing information about the etiology of mental disorders. The diagnoses, however, are composed of descrip-
tive criteria that are intended to be silent on etiology. In fact, the Introduction
to the DSM states absolutely nothing about causation. The way we clinicians
and researchers usually think about these categories—as in mood disorders,
for example—is not as *a syndrome we call depression*, but rather as *a syndrome
caused by depression*.

Beyond a few organic disorders covered by the DSM, most diagnoses in
the manual do not have known causes, pathophysiology, or investigational
technologies to confirm them. Arguably, the most common mental disorders
causing the greatest burden of disease worldwide, such as mood disorders,
have frustrated our attempts at elucidating their pathophysiology or even developing objective investigational tools that assist in verifying the absence or
presence of the diagnosis. For the most part, the best we can do is ask specific
questions that have a high sensitivity at picking up the presence of significant
symptoms. Therefore, several of the key factors that support the primacy of
diagnosis in the rest of health care do not yet apply to mental health diagnoses.

Unfortunately, the prevalence and use of the traditional medical model for
mental disorders are problematic given that the nosology consists of diagnoses that do not satisfy the criteria for validity.[3,11-14] The complexity of
mental disorders and absence of their verifiability appear to provide a blank
canvas upon which individuals and societies freely draw simplistic and specious formulations. Consequently, we need to consider both the utility of the
current diagnostic framework and how it is used.

This does not mean, however, that the DSM is useless. Far from it. As per
Kendell and Jablensky,[10] we can use the DSM to help us more completely
identify client symptoms, leading to fuller diagnostic impressions and, ultimately, comprehensive treatment targets. To achieve this requires a blending
of other emerging approaches to mental health care. We elaborate on this idea
in Chapter 7.

DSM-5 and the Biopsychosocial Model

In the DSM-5, the authors' acceptance of the limited validity and specificity
of the DSM's framework expressed in the Introduction gives way in the Use
of the Manual section to a self-assured tone regarding its utility. Despite the
absence of any diagnostic criteria related to formulation, and the authors'
acknowledgments that the DSM does not address causation and treatment, formulation is touted as critical to both: "It requires clinical training

to recognize when the combination of predisposing, precipitating, perpetu-ating, and protective factors has resulted in a psychopathological condition in which physical signs and symptoms exceed normal ranges" (p. 19).[3] This assertion about the continuing importance of Engel's biopsychosocial model, published in 1977, implies that a causal pathway can be found by using it.[15] This is completely at odds with the fact that we don't know the causes of any common mental disorder. We view this thinking as problematic, particularly if we accept the absence of absolute validity of diagnoses and the lack of ev-idence supporting the commonly used biopsychosocial model of formula-tion.[16-19] In addition, there are many other criticisms that have been leveled at Engel's model, and some of these consist of the view that it is eclectic, circular, overinclusive, simplistic, unscientific while purporting to be scientific, not humanistic (attempts to incorporate psychology and social sciences versus humanities), does not allow for prioritization of treatment, and conflates cau-sation and management.[20,21] McLaren argues that the biopsychosocial model is not a model at all because it does not emerge from a well-developed theory of mind and as a model has no predictive value:

> Unless there is an integrating theory already in place, gathering biological, psy-chological and sociological data about people will only yield scattered lumps of information which don't relate to each other in any coherent sense. Without an over-arching theory to integrate the fields from which the data derive, associations between differing classes of information are meaningless. (p. 277)[18]

How are we to accept the suggestion that *causal formulation* is critical to treatment when it is mental disorder nosologies and their diagnostic templates that determine research and guidelines related to treatment? There seems to be a cavernous expanse between the rhetoric surrounding formula-tion and the scientific support of its utility in achieving desired outcomes. We seek explanatory models for patients' suffering that often lead us to premature speculation, bias, or anchor us in specious hypotheses as immutable facts. We can never disprove these narratives because they are retrospective, anecdotal, and based on opaque interpretations.

Similarly, there are many criticisms that can be and have been leveled at the DSM and the multiple revisions since its inception in 1952. It is impor-tant to note that for all its problems, we need to appreciate that thousands of clinicians and scientists have had input into its various iterations as they have worked to try to classify mental disorders in a way that is coherent and par-simonious. It is, however, in our opinion, a Frankenstein's monster, requiring continual re-creation. As such, it is a reflection on its makers rather than on the poor monster itself. The attempt to adjudicate inclusions, exclusions, and categorization on a combination of limited science and interest groups gives rise to profound limitations and impedes unbiased progress. The current iteration of the manual states that

> despite the problems posed by categorical diagnoses . . . it is premature scientifically to propose alternative definitions for most disorders. The organizational structure is meant to serve as a bridge to new diagnostic approaches without disrupting current clinical practice or research. (p. 13)[3]

The DSM-5 task force is referring to the use of a *dimensional* approach to the classification of mental disorders to deal with some of the difficulties inherent to the nosology. An important barrier to changing it is the extent to which the DSM is embedded in so many aspects of mental health, including clinician training, research, funding, physician billing, organizational statistics, insurance coverage, medical legal issues, clinical treatments, communication between clinicians, communication between clinicians and patients, how people define themselves and others, and even within common parlance.

We can well imagine how difficult and disruptive it would be to significantly alter this nosology or to develop an alternative approach to organizing mental illness, its assessment and management. This is an example of the *sunk cost bias*. Simply defined, this bias reflects the tendency that the more we invest in something, the more difficult it is to walk away from it even when it is a losing venture.[22] Beyond deepening our losses, this pattern of thinking also delays learning from failures and exploring alternative approaches. The sunk cost bias in health care is especially damaging because it impedes progress by wasting resources and delaying the pursuit of novel approaches.

Utility and Limitations of the Diagnostic Frame

What, then, is the clinical utility of mental disorder diagnoses in the absence of known pathophysiology or specific treatments? By utility, we are also referring to the degree to which a diagnosis assists in mitigating the risk of harm to self or others, disability, and degree of suffering. This is an essential question to ask because of the axiom that an accurate diagnosis is critical to effective health care.

In 2015, the National Academies of Sciences, Engineering, and Medicine released an excellent report on improving diagnosis in health care. The report identified diagnostic error as a priority and stated the following sin the Preface: "The correct diagnosis is a critical aspect of healthcare" (p. xiii).[5] It did not, however, go on to state that interventions can only begin when an accurate diagnosis has been ascertained.

In most areas of medicine other than psychiatry, diagnoses come complete with known causes, pathophysiology, history, physical signs, investigations, treatments, and prognosis. Such diagnoses are useful nosologically, and they are clinically efficient when accurate. Even for illness with completely delineated pathophysiology, however, an accurate diagnosis may not be sufficient to guide comprehensive management at every stage of treatment. For instance, a patient arrives at the emergency department in respiratory distress—several life-saving interventions may need to be initiated in a time window that closes before an accurate diagnosis has been confirmed. Delay the treatment and you may be left with nothing but postmortem investigations to delineate the contributing diagnoses. Consider the recent COVID-19 pandemic and the need to manage respiratory distress before all investigations can be completed. Even testing positive for the COVID-19 virus is insufficient to explain a person's health status given the profound variations in the course of illness within populations and the role of comorbidities. Similarly, in managing mental health, risks of harm, impairment, and suffering may need to be addressed before clinicians are able to achieve clarity on possible diagnoses.

In addition to the difficulty of establishing a single mental disorder diagnosis, comorbid diagnoses (as a concept) are common in health care. When, in the early 1980s, it appeared that multiple DSM diagnoses commonly co-occur, it was also called *comorbidity*, denoting the simultaneous co-occurrence of two distinct disorders (e.g., a stomach virus and arthritis). By the time it was realized that *co-occurring* mental disorders were rarely discrete, the term comorbidity had come to be used so frequently that it stuck, to the point that even authors who have roundly criticized its use continue to use the term.[23–25] We argue that the idea of comorbidity in the case of the DSM is an indicator of an imperfect classification system that requires a means for accounting for the presence of similar or different phenomena (signs, symptoms, and behaviors) when seeking parsimony regarding a diagnosis.

This all points toward a significant likelihood that mental disorders are rarely distinct entities. Nonetheless, comprehensive diagnostic assessments that incorporate the SCID only find more than one diagnosis in approximately 45% of cases.[26] Several studies of diagnostic practice-as-usual have found that clinicians fail to identify numerous co-occurring disorders that are relatively discreet, uncommon, or on a particular spectrum, and that the catch-all diagnosis of adjustment disorder is more frequently made.[27–29] Regardless of whether we interpret the results as indicative of discrete conditions, concluding that multiple diagnoses in a single individual are an artifact of the

DSM is simplistic. At minimum, the identification of extensive and diverse symptoms in presentations is representative of greater complexity, worse outcomes, and that the individual is at risk of greater impairment in several spheres of life.[28,29]

To reiterate, we need to remember that diagnosis of a mental disorder does not provide us with an explanation of its underlying process. However, the American Psychiatric Association's (APA) website states,

> DSM-5 is a manual for assessment and diagnosis of mental disorders and does not include information or guidelines for treatment of any disorder. That said, determining an accurate diagnosis is the first step toward being able to appropriately treat any medical condition, and mental disorders are no exception.[30]

Note that the APA has gone beyond the National Academies of Sciences, Engineering, and Medicine's assertion that diagnoses are "critical" by stating that a diagnosis is "the first step" to treatment. Ironically, the statement is that "an accurate diagnosis is the first step." Diagnostic accuracy in mental health is elusive and impossible to confirm or refute. What would this mean for treatment if the APA's statement were true and followed?

Given the prevalence of the DSM's use, and the place it holds in terms of how we organize our thinking around mental disorders and their management, we think it is essential to look at how the DSM relates to risk of harm and its management.

DSM as a Cognitive Organizing Tool

The DSM allows us to chunk information and provides a common language that clinicians and researchers can use to speak to each other, third-party payors, government organizations, and patients and their families. It also allows us to organize our thinking and provides a description and listing of phenomena (symptoms and signs) and how these may co-occur. Whether intended or not, the nosology also informs treatment plans, research, and clinical funding and the epidemiology of these diseases.[31]

So how might our nosology assist us in negotiating uncertainty? Consider the following ways it helps reduce our cognitive load when we are trying to assess a patient:

- It assists clinicians to manage complexity by parsing out information.
- It provides a finite set of conditions to consider.

- It demonstrates that some symptoms present in recognizable patterns.
- It contains information on risk and functional impairments, and it assists with differential diagnoses.

There are, however, several characteristics of the DSM criteria that are themselves imbued with uncertainty as well as missing important information for assessment and management. For example, the language used is vague, such as "most days" or "most of the day." The most common risks of harm associated with each diagnosis are not specified. Diagnostic criteria do not assist in gauging the changing phases of illness. Impairment is not defined or contrasted with the range of normal by using discrete criteria or suggesting levels of impairment for differing degrees of severity of an illness. Some impairments associated with specific conditions are identified in general terms with limited utility. Last, the DSM does not address the degree of suffering or necessarily the nature of the distress that may be associated with each diagnosis. It is one thing to know what we are calling a disorder, and it is quite another thing to guide its management.

If the DSM is to be more useful, we think it is essential to make overt the uncertainty associated with diagnosis and how to mitigate it., It should provide clinicians with more and explicit information about risk of harm, disability, and distress associated with each diagnosis. The DSM should go beyond listing diagnoses independently or on spectrums and address common comorbidities as clusters requiring special consideration and identifying risk of harm and disability with such clusters.

The DSM and ICD are nonetheless considered useful taxonomies that organize phenomena into a manageable number of syndromes and provide frameworks for further testing, debate, and communication. But are they? For instance, in establishing a diagnosis of major depressive disorder, the DSM criteria can be organized into a staggering number of combinations that would be impossible for clinicians to appreciate. Eiko Fried calculated that "there are up to 10,377 ways to qualify for a diagnosis of major depression (alone), but there are up to 341,737 ways to qualify for a diagnosis of melancholia, which is a subtype of depression."[31] This applies to the other diagnoses in the manual as well. If we have more than 10,000 combinations that can be called depression, this begs the question whether we are dealing with a well-defined and delineated entity—especially when all the combinations will inevitably overlap with other DSM diagnoses and thus increase the objective uncertainty exponentially.

History has shown that the diagnostic taxonomy in psychiatry and psychology is not fixed, although it is very slow to change. This pace of change is in itself a reflection of unwarranted certainty in its constructs and their imperviousness to being verified or falsified. The DSM has been so resistant to change that cultural change has outpaced it. For example, in 1973, 5,854 psychiatrists voted to remove homosexuality from the DSM and 3,810 voted to retain it. The APA compromised and renamed it sexual disorientation disturbance. It wasn't until 1987 that "homosexuality" was removed from the manual as a psychopathology. And it was not until 1992 that it was removed from WHO ICD-10.[32] The pathologizing of sexual orientation is now characterized as prejudicial, oppressive, and more, but it was also a spectacular error that reflects the vulnerability of the nosology to feckless theories and pseudoscience. Karl Popper's assertion, made in the 1950s, that theories must be falsifiable to be considered scientific continues to exclude almost every theory and diagnosis contained within the DSM.[33]

Despite the lesson of "homosexuality," we continue to consider phenomena related to gender as pathological and have included issues related to gender identity within the DSM-5 under the name "gender dysphoria." The rationale provided reflects currently changing norms, along with the degree of suffering experienced, but also the centrality of diagnosis within Western health care systems. The APA explains its rationale as follows:

> Persons experiencing gender dysphoria need a diagnostic term that protects their access to care and won't be used against them in social, occupational, or legal areas. When it comes to access to care, many of the treatment options for this condition include counseling, cross-sex hormones, gender reassignment surgery, and social and legal transition to the desired gender. To get insurance coverage for the medical treatments, individuals need a diagnosis. The Sexual and Gender Identity Disorders Work Group was concerned that removing the condition as a psychiatric diagnosis—as some had suggested—would jeopardize access to care.[34]

A nosology that conflates syndromes and politics compromises its scientific credibility.

In Praise of a Phenomenological Approach

A more transparent approach would be to attach probabilities of certitude to diagnoses, but the current state of empirical knowledge does not yet allow clinicians to do this reliably. The safest approach would be to use the DSM to guide pattern recognition, recognize our inherent vulnerability to error, and continuously examine the diagnosis as the hypothesis that it is. Unfortunately, this is not how we are trained.

Independent of diagnostic categorization and criteria, phenomena associated with mental disorders are less influenced by our pragmatic need to classify. Despite the challenges in eliciting, identifying, and confirming the said phenomena, we can at least be more confident that they exist in nature. Furthermore, we can identify phenomena independent of a determined diagnosis. A pitfall related to diagnostic closure is that we fail to recognize or look for phenomena of overlapping and unrecognized diagnoses. This is directly tied to anchoring and confirmation bias. To state it logically, phenomena are not dependent on diagnosis though diagnosis is dependent on phenomena. The clinician's observations and assessment of phenomena will invariably be influenced by the differential diagnoses that arise in their minds. This brings to mind the adage that what is looked for is what is seen. This is discussed further in Chapter 5, in which we compare the relative performance of clinicians using structured assessments to practice as usual.

Most of the currently available mental health treatments target phenomena more accurately than diagnoses. This makes sense given that pharmacological and psychological treatments are directed at signs and symptoms. For instance, we use dopaminergic antagonists in the treatment of hallucinations and delusions regardless of the diagnosis. Even more to the point, we use second-generation antipsychotics in the treatment of major depressive disorder, bipolar affective disorder, Tourette's syndrome, obsessive–compulsive disorder (OCD), and many dementias. We use serotonergic specific re-uptake inhibitors for mood disorders, anxiety disorders, schizoaffective disorders, personality disorders, premature ejaculation, eating disorders, and so on. We look forward to a future in which the nonspecificity of pharmacologic treatments gives way to effective pharmacotherapy or other biological treatments that are specific to discrete mental disorders. To date, no pharmacological treatment that is specific and exclusive to a singular mental disorder has been arrived at by design or serendipity. The same can be said about our psychological treatments. They are all transdiagnostic or phenomenological, although they may not be labeled as such. For example, we have cognitive–behavioral therapy (CBT) for OCD, social phobia, depression, psychosis, and so on. With some minor variations, CBT is the vehicle being used. Innovative approaches to psychological treatments with transdiagnostic applicability are in the process of development and testing. The Unified Protocol for Transdiagnostic Treatment of Emotional Disorders is a modular treatment approach to mental disorders that does just that: It incorporates elements common to several psychotherapies and is intended for use with a variety of mental disorders. These modules cultivate such skills as mindfulness, cognitive flexibility, the reduction of experiential avoidance, increased distress tolerance, and interoceptive emotion-focused exposure. Although there is limited evidence supporting this approach, results are promising.[35]

So, if no diagnostic-specific treatments exist, why should clinical care be predicated upon specific diagnoses? The advantage of nonspecific interventions is that clinicians can proceed with treatment predicated upon phenomena while continuing to test diagnostic hypotheses. The disadvantage is that this can mask diagnostic errors and reinforce unwarranted certainty because treatment response is often interpreted as a function of diagnostic accuracy. This perception is tautological and grown from the same ground that confuses the criteria for a major depressive episode as symptoms *caused by depression.*

Summary

In this chapter, we discussed features of mental disorder nosology that relate to uncertainty in diagnosis and management. Considering the enormous gaps in the current understanding of the brain, mind, and related mental disorders, it is inevitable that the nosology is incomplete and otherwise limited. At the level of its most basic aim of facilitating the use of common language, so that clinicians, researchers and others are reliably referring to the same entity, the evidence suggests that current nosologies are also failing. A concrete view into this failure is provided by studies of clinician error and/or agreement in diagnosing mental disorders. In Chapter 5, we provide a glimpse into this fascinating literature.

References

1. World Health Organization. International Classification of Diseases (ICD) information sheet. https://www.who.int/classifications/icd/factsheet/en. Accessed April 26, 2020.
2. World Health Organization. *International Classification of Diseases.* 11th rev. World Health Organization; 2018. https://www.who.int/classifications/icd/en. Accessed April 26, 2020.
3. American Psychiatric Association. *Diagnostic and statistical manual of mental disorders.* 5th ed. American Psychiatric Publishing; 2013.
4. Sartorius N, Kaelber CT, Cooper JE, et al. Progress toward achieving a common language in psychiatry: Results from the field trial of the clinical guidelines accompanying the WHO classification of mental and behavioral disorders in ICD-10. *Arch Gen Psychiatry.* 1993;50(2):115–124.

5. National Academies of Sciences, Engineering, and Medicine. *Improving Diagnosis in Health Care*. National Academies Press; 2015.
6. Walfish S, McAlister B, O'Donnell P, Lambert MJ. An investigation of self-assessment bias in mental health providers. *Psychol Rep*. 2012;110(2):639–644.
7. Smith JD, Dumont F. Confidence in psychodiagnosis: What makes us so sure? *Clin Psychol Psychother*. 2002;9(4):292–298.
8. Miller DJ, Spengler ES, Spengler PM. A meta-analysis of confidence and judgment accuracy in clinical decision making. *J Couns Psychol*. 2015;62(4):553–567.
9. Desmarais SL, Nicholls TL, Read JD, Brink J. Confidence and accuracy in assessments of short-term risks presented by forensic psychiatric patients. *J Forensic Psychiatry Psychol*. 2010;21(1):1–22.
10. Kendell R, Jablensky A. Distinguishing between the validity and utility of psychiatric diagnoses. *Am J Psychiatry*. 2003;160(1):4–12.
11. Vanheule S, Desmet M, Meganck R, et al. Reliability in psychiatric diagnosis with the DSM: Old wine in new barrels. *Psychother Psychosom*. 2014;83(5):313–314.
12. Kendler KS, Zachar P, Craver C. What kinds of things are psychiatric disorders? *Psychol Med*. 2011;41(6):1143–1150.
13. Kendler KS. DSM disorders and their criteria: How should they inter-relate? *Psychol Med*. 2017;47(12):2054–2060.
14. Park SC, Kim JM, Jun TY, et al. How many different symptom combinations fulfil the diagnostic criteria for major depressive disorder? Results from the CRESCEND study. *Nord J Psychiatry*. 2017;71(3):217–222.
15. Engel GL. The need for a new medical model: a challenge for biomedicine. *Science*. 1977;196(4286):129–136.
16. Lehman BJ, David DM, Gruber JA. Rethinking the biopsychosocial model of health: Understanding health as a dynamic system. *Social Personality Psychol Compass*. 2017;11(8):e12328.
17. McLaren N. A critical review of the biopsychosocial model. *Aust N Z J Psychiatry*. 1998;32(1):86–92.
18. McLaren N. The myth of the biopsychosocial model. *Aust N Z J Psychiatry*. 2006;40(3):277–278.
19. Ghaemi SN. The biopsychosocial model in psychiatry: A critique. *Am J Psychiatry*. 2011;121:451–457.
20. Benning TB. Limitations of the biopsychosocial model in psychiatry. *Adv Med Educ Pract*. 2015;6:347–352.
21. Arkes HR, Blumer C. The psychology of sunk cost. *Organ Behav Hum Decis Process*. 1985;35(1):124–140.
22. Waldman ID, Lilienfeld SO. Applications of taxometric methods to problems of comorbidity: Perspectives and challenges. *Clin Psychol Sci Pract*. 2001;8(4):520–527.
23. Lilienfeld SO. Comorbidity between and within childhood externalizing and internalizing disorders: Reflections and directions. *J Abnorm Child Psychol*. 2003;31(3):285–291.
24. Lilienfeld SO, Waldman ID, Israel AC. A critical examination of the use of the term and concept of comorbidity in psychopathology research. *Clin Psychol Sci Pract*. 1994;1(1):71–83.
25. Pitman A, Tyrer P. Implementing clinical guidelines for self harm—highlighting key issues arising from the NICE guideline for self-harm. *Psychol Psychother*. 2008;81(Pt 4):377–397.
26. Zimmerman M, Mattia JI. Psychiatric diagnosis in clinical practice: Is comorbidity being missed? *Compr Psychiatry*. 1999;40(3):182–191.
27. Zimmerman M. A review of 20 years of research on overdiagnosis and underdiagnosis in the Rhode Island Methods to Improve Diagnostic Assessment and Services (MIDAS) project. *Can J Psychiatry*. 2016;61(2):71–79.

28. Shear MK, Greeno C, Kang J, et al. Diagnosis of nonpsychotic patients in community clinics. *Am J Psychiatry.* 2000;157(4):581–587.
29. Avasthi A, Sarkar S, Grover S. Approaches to psychiatric nosology: A viewpoint. *Indian J Psychiatry.* 2014;56(3):301–304.
30. American Psychiatric Association. DSM-5 frequently asked questions. https://www. psychiatry.org/psychiatrists/practice/dsm/feedback-and-questions/frequently-asked-questions. Accessed January 2020.
31. Fried E. 10,377 ways for major depression, but 341,737 ways for melancholia. https://eiko-fried.com/10377-ways-for-major-depression-but-341737-ways-for-melancholia; 2018.
32. Drescher J. Out of DSM: Depathologizing homosexuality. *Behav Sci.* 2015;5(4):565–575.
33. Popper K. *The Logic of Scientific Discovery.* 2nd ed. Routledge; 2002.
34. AmericanPsychiatricAssociation.Genderdysphoria.https://www.psychiatry.org.Published 2013. https://r.search.yahoo.com/_ylt=AwrE1xja2NhgMgoAF_hXNyoA;_ylu =Y29sbwNiZjEEcG9zAzEEdnRpZANDMTYxMl8xBHNlYwNzcg--/RV=2/ RE=1624852827/RO=10/RU=https%3a%2f%2fwww.psychiatry.org%2fFile%2520Libra ry%2fPsychiatrists%2fPractice%2fDSM%2fAPA_DSM-5-Gender-Dysphoria.pdf/RK= 2/RS=HGdZevgg1ZIvo5Qtzhc4Y8HDtFE-
35. Barlow DH, Farchione TJ, Bullis JR, et al. The unified protocol for transdiagnostic treatment of emotional disorders compared with diagnosis-specific protocols for anxiety disorders: A randomized clinical trial. *JAMA Psychiatry.* 2017;74(9):875–884.

5
Diagnostic Errors in Practice

Having discussed some aspects of the *Diagnostic and Statistical Manual of Mental Disorders* (DSM) that may contribute to unwarranted certainty in its users, this chapter explores the diagnostic error in mental health.

As discussed previously, objective methods of verifying or falsifying diagnoses of mental disorders do not currently exist. Consequently, it is the reliability, completeness, and accuracy of the information gathered in mental health assessments, combined with the "correct" application of the DSM criteria, that currently determine whether diagnoses are accurate. Only after sorting through the ways in which the assessment data can be combined does the task become a relatively simple matter of thinking through the 157 sets of diagnostic criteria and their overlaps. The fragility of the information sources, the ambiguity of the information itself, and the changing nature of mental disorders require repeating this process iteratively as information is corrected, eliminated, or added over time—repetition that is rare in actual practice.

Errors are inevitable in such a process, especially errors of omission. These are evident in several steps of a diagnostic assessment. For instance, the frequency with which clinicians do not elicit the full extent of a client's symptoms is then reflected in the failure to list all the diagnoses that a patient's presentation satisfies. We are not simply referring to a differential diagnosis but, rather, to a complete list of DSM diagnoses whose criteria are met by the elicited symptoms. So, what actually constitutes an error?

Defining Diagnostic Error—It's More Difficult Than You Think

The National Academies of Sciences, Engineering, and Medicine's report on diagnostic error included a review of the world's literature, collaboration with international experts, and broad stakeholder input.[1] Such rigorous thinking on this issue was unprecedented. The report's authors examined existing definitions of diagnostic error from throughout the world and, recognizing the need for improvement, suggested a new one. Based on its relative simplicity, clarity, and applicability to equitable health care systems, we have adopted their definition. They define diagnostic error as "the failure to (a) establish an accurate and timely explanation of the patient's health problem(s) or (b) communicate that explanation to the patient."[1] Note that this definition incorporates the user's perspective; thus, failure to communicate the diagnosis also constitutes a diagnostic error.[1]

At first glance, we were overcome by an urge to quibble with the communication component of the definition. Surely, a diagnosis is correct regardless of whether it is communicated. Yet, no clinician would argue with the importance of obtaining a patient's informed consent before initiating treatment. A patient or delegate, however, cannot provide informed consent without information about the diagnosis to which the treatment options pertain. If there is to be no intervention, a diagnosis has no treatment to guide. If a diagnosis arises in a clinical setting without affecting management, it is a dud. Ergo, failure to communicate a diagnosis is a diagnostic error.

In reference to the degree of certainty in diagnoses and its relationship to patient communication, the report discusses that communicating a diagnosis to a patient in a timely manner will be dependent on the time it takes to arrive at an explanation for the patient's symptoms. One suggestion to manage this is that the clinicians transparently share with the patient the degree of certainty regarding the diagnosis or explanation of the condition. We add that the substantial probability of diagnostic error (an essential aspect of full disclosure) should be woven into all risk:benefit discussions when engaging patients in informed consent. This might give clinicians pause to reflect on their level of confidence in their surmised diagnoses.

Nonetheless, it is our opinion that the definition suggested by the National Academies of Sciences, Engineering, and Medicine warrants a closer inspection. To begin with, what does it mean for a diagnosis to be *accurate*? The report attempts to explain such accuracy as follows: "A diagnosis is not accurate if it differs from the true condition a patient has (or does not have) or if it is imprecise and incomplete (lacking in sufficient detail)" (p. 85).[1]

Scrutinizing the definition at this level reveals the factors that confound the translation of the definition into practice. To begin with, the *accuracy* of a diagnosis is judged by comparison to *the true condition*. But how and by whom is *the true condition* established, particularly in mental disorders? In many instances, this is not possible, and the fuzzy margins of uncertainty surrounding diagnostic errors make agreement on a specific error difficult. We all agree errors are made in general. We, however, often disagree when we have made one. The solution has been to establish a low threshold by which a diagnosis is considered correct and a high threshold for a diagnosis to be considered wrong. All of this means that research into diagnostic error likely underestimates how often we are wrong in our diagnostic judgments.

Other Definitions of Diagnostic Error

Highlighting the lack of agreement around what constitutes a diagnostic error, we consider other definitions. Mark Graber defines it as a "diagnosis that was unintentionally delayed (sufficient information was available earlier), wrong (another diagnosis was made before the correct one), or missed (no diagnosis was ever made), as judged from the eventual appreciation of more definitive information" (p. 82).[2] By suggesting that a determination of error will be predicated upon "eventual appreciation of more definitive information (p. 82)," Graber reminds us that most diagnoses are made by clinicians without the benefit of complete and accurate information. Nowhere is this more obvious than in mental health, in which conditions evolve, making it difficult to ascertain if a diagnosis is *correct* in one moment and then *wrong* at another. Current training, however, fails to prevent clinicians from mistaking the diagnostic process in mental health as a singular, one-time event. It is difficult for us to remember that diagnoses are human tools, not nature's rules.

Disagreement Between Assessment Methods: Uncertainty or Error

We can begin to disentangle the relative contribution of irreducible uncertainty inherent to assessing mental disorders by starting with a basic premise. If I as a clinician fail to ask the necessary questions from all sources, consequently not eliciting the full complement of features of a mental disorder, then any diagnostic error could be due to my incomplete method of assessment. In contrast, if a clinician does a complete assessment, including screening questions for the more inconspicuous or ambiguous disorders in the presentation, then the error may result primarily from the objective uncertainty intrinsic to mental disorders and the limitations of available assessment methods. Obviously, objective uncertainty and assessment methods interact to contribute to error. We have some control over assessment methods, including the extent to which we employ them over time, but none on the irreducible uncertainties. How might we manage this operationally? The first step is recognizing the inescapable susceptibility to error and utilizing a rigorous, prospective approach to assessment that reduces methodological influence on assessment errors—for instance, failing to obtain available information or failing to consider all possible diagnoses. This translates into the use of structured assessments.

There are two broad categories of structure as applied to assessment. One is the simple use of scales or questionnaires in conjunction with an unstructured or semistructured interview. The other is the use of a structured interview such as the Structured Clinical Interview for DSM (SCID) or the Mini International Neuropsychiatric Interview (MINI). One question that we explore is whether any level of structure improves assessment accuracy and what the relationship might be between the degree of structure and diagnostic errors.

Client satisfaction or acceptance of methods is important because we depend on rapport to foster trust so that people share their thoughts, emotions, and behaviors to inform assessment. Many clinicians express concern that structured assessments are robotic, miss nuances arising from unstructured interviews, and that clients do not like them. In addition, a common criticism of structured assessments is that they identify superfluous diagnoses that are disconnected from patient concerns. We have selected studies that address these important concerns.

How Frequent Are Diagnostic Errors in Mental Health Care?

We have previously drawn an analogy with meteorologists. It does not come as a shock to most of us when our weekend plans are washed out by rain contrary to the week's weather reports. Most of us, however, are in disbelief when we are informed, or realize, that we have made a diagnostic error. At minimum, most of us would like to believe that clinicians' diagnostic accuracy must outperform meteorological predictions, but it doesn't. The numerous studies comparing diagnostic methods and agreement enable reasonable conclusions about diagnostic accuracy in most clinical settings. We have selected several that are particularly informative in illuminating the frequency of diagnostic error.

Raymond Kotwicki and Philip Harvey published results of a 3-year study evaluating the influence of structured assessment methods on DSM diagnoses in a community psychiatric rehabilitation setting.[3] Using the staff of a community treatment program, they evaluated the effect of training staff to independently conduct diagnostic assessments using the SCID for DSM-IV and the MINI. The results of the structured assessments were compared to practice as usual in 313 cases.

The study's primary focus was to compare the stability of diagnoses from admission to discharge across three different methods of assessment over treatment periods averaging 13 weeks. Referral source diagnoses, in addition to unstructured admission assessment by the study's raters, were compared to the diagnoses made using the SCID and MINI. The reported findings were statistically significant and not subtle. Admission diagnoses derived from unstructured assessments were changed 74% of the time. In comparison, only 4% of SCID and 11% of MINI diagnoses were changed. Some specific diagnoses provided by referring clinicians were especially prone to error. Diagnoses of schizoaffective disorder were changed in approximately 90% of cases upon assessment by the SCID or MINI.

As we know, "managed care companies are often interested in matching treatments to diagnoses and may refuse to reimburse for treatments that are not approved for specific indications, suggesting that in order to offer suitable treatments to patients accurate diagnosis is important" (p. 15).[3] This puts pressure on the clinician to arrive at a diagnosis regardless of accuracy to ensure reimbursement. However, as we have outlined, accuracy of diagnosis is problematic, and a focus on managing risk of harm, disability, and suffering would enable treatment to proceed pending clarification of diagnosis.

It is important to note that although time-consuming (an argument often used against their use), the superiority of structured diagnostic assessment methods compared with usual practice is considerably greater than that of one antidepressant over another or one structured psychotherapy over another. Professionally, most regulatory bodies would not countenance a clinician's assertion that psychosis is best treated with exercise alone. Yet, we accept clinicians continuing to use methods of diagnostic assessment that are no more accurate than a coin toss.

Kotwicki and Harvey conclude that multiple stakeholders would benefit from the use of structured diagnostic assessment at the time of admission to more intensive settings.[3] We believe the benefit to be even broader in its potential. Whether it is the changing landscape of symptoms as mental disorders evolve or as updated information is collected prospectively, the fluctuating nature of presentations suggests that all assessments in every context would benefit from structured methods. Structured diagnostic assessment should be considered an ongoing process.

The enormous ocean of peer-reviewed publications hides pearls in places that are typically outside popular view. From the *Journal of Correctional*

Health Care comes such a pearl.[4] A group from the University of Ottawa in Canada reviewed the international literature on diagnostic error in the assessment of mental disorders in correctional facilities. The review included a study conducted in France.[5]

A key aspect of Falissard et al.'s study was that each inmate was assessed by two clinicians both present simultaneously.[5] Consequently, the clinicians were exposed to the same responses to questions, observable behaviors, and other information that emerged during the assessment. Assessments were 2 hours in length. Prior to any discussion between the clinician duo, each independently documented their diagnoses. The authors calculated the level of diagnostic agreement between them. To reduce the probability of being led astray by a false level of agreement reflected in a simple percentage, the study applied a statistical formula used by most diagnostic agreement studies. The most common statistic used is the Cohen's kappa, which for nonstatisticians translates a kappa value to a percentage. We have, for ease of discussion, translated the kappa into an error rate shown in Table 5.1.

Table 5.1 illustrates a subset of the diagnoses reported by Falissard et al.,[5] including those with the lowest and highest levels of agreement. When we remember that these figures represent agreement between a series of two clinicians in the same interview, at the same time, using the same data, the level of agreement is not reassuring.

On the one hand, it could be argued that a 91% agreement in diagnosing a condition such as alcohol dependence is impressive, but the clinical implications of a 9% error rate needs to be considered more thoughtfully. Let us take a relatively simple example, such as alcohol dependence, and think

Table 5.1 Diagnostic Agreement Between a Series of Two Clinicians in the Same Interview

Diagnosis	Cohen's Kappa	Error Rate (%)
Schizophrenia	0.64	36
Bipolar disorders	0.68	32
Panic disorder	0.76	24
Psychotic disorders	0.76	24
Generalized anxiety	0.77	23
Post-traumatic stress disorder	0.78	22
Major depressive disorders	0.87	13
Alcohol dependence	0.91	9
Drug dependence	0.95	5

Adapted from Falissard et al.[5]

about the consequences of missing the diagnosis (an error). Focusing on material risk exclusively, this translates into a delay in identifying, or completely missing, a change in mental status as potential signs of alcohol withdrawal. This would lead to a failure to treat the individual in a timely manner and increase the risk of client mortality and morbidity as well as institutional liability.

Based on both Falissard et al.'s study and their overall review of the literature, Martin and co-authors defined a diagnostic error in their forensic context as "any inmate whose diagnostic classification varies depending on the method of arriving at this classification" (p. 110).[4] This brings us to a key principle in diagnosis that is hidden by the language of an *opinion* when referring to a clinician's diagnosis, especially when it is found to be wrong. "It was my opinion at the time" is an especially common phrase used by clinicians heard in malpractice proceedings. Where there is diagnostic disagreement, there is diagnostic error.

Accuracy requires a complete identification of all diagnoses informed by the patient's presentation regardless of whether clinicians view them as a comorbidity or an artifact of overlapping criteria. This is a critical point in the diagnosis of mental disorders because the DSM lists syndromes, not discrete diseases whose overlap can be disentangled using objective measures that penetrate deeper than symptoms. Differing diagnoses are not simply matters of opinion; it means one or both clinicians have made an error, and this affects client outcomes.

MIDAS

A group in Rhode Island, USA, led by Mark Zimmerman has been diligently working to improve diagnostic assessment in an outpatient setting since the 1990s. By the time of a 2016 review, his team had assessed approximately 3,800 persons using the DSM-IV SCID in addition to a battery of other structured assessments in a community outpatient setting.[6] We would be remiss in writing a chapter exploring diagnostic accuracy in mental health care without including this team's work.

Zimmerman's research uses naturalistic methods that are applicable to any clinician working in any setting. In 1994, Zimmerman and his team began the Rhode Island Methods to Improve Diagnostic Assessment and Services (MIDAS) project that integrates clinical research with routine clinical practice. In one of their reports published in 1999, they focused on the identification of psychiatric comorbidity in persons referred to a general outpatient psychiatry clinic at Rhode Island Hospital in Providence, Rhode Island.[6] The study compared the identification of comorbidity elicited by structured diagnostic assessment with unstructured, usual practice.

Patients were given a choice between undergoing a routine assessment or a comprehensive one. The routine assessments conducted by the clinic's psychologists and psychiatrists were the typical 45–60 minutes, including the time spent synthesizing findings into a consultation report. In contrast, the group of patients assessed comprehensively benefited from a 3-hour assessment, following which the clinicians devoted 3 hours to preparing a detailed report. Despite the limits to interpreting group differences, the findings reported are consistent with others in which structured assessments identify a greater number and variety of diagnoses versus practice as usual. One of the reassuring aspects of this study is its applicability to real-world clinical settings. The patients were unsolicited referrals to an actual outpatient service rather than patients specifically recruited for research purposes. Patients undergoing routine assessments were evaluated by experienced staff psychologists and psychiatrists. Other clinicians were specifically hired and intensively trained to conduct comprehensive structured assessments on the group of patients choosing this approach. The latter patients were assessed using structured methods, including the Structured Clinical Interview for DSM-IV Axis I Disorders, along with other interview tools. A psychiatrist reviewed each patient and report before finalizing the diagnoses. The number of people assessed by each assessment method was large relative to most diagnosis studies, with 500 individuals per group.

Before sharing Zimmerman's findings, it is helpful to summarize the background on mental disorder comorbidity. Formally structured assessments identify more than one disorder twice as often as unstructured assessments. Translating this pattern into the language of diagnostic errors, when clinicians do not utilize available structured methods of assessment, they double the number of mistakes they make in diagnosis. At minimum, the findings suggest that unstructured assessments underestimate the degree of complexity in patient presentations. This perspective aligns with current opinions regarding human judgment, that our cognition tends to ignore complexity. Heuristics, for instance, are cognitive strategies that simplify complex information for the purpose of rapid judgments but at the cost of decreased accuracy and increased error.

It is difficult to resist reiterating a frequent criticism of structured assessments offered by many clinicians: "I find that structured assessments limit my ability to appreciate the full complexity of the person in front of me." There would certainly be merit in the criticism if a structured assessment exclusively utilized questions relating to diagnostic criteria. The implication is that structured assessments do not add anything to the current standard of practice and that structured assessments impact negatively on rapport. Zimmerman's description of the depth and breadth of the structured assessments conducted, and patients' positive experiences with them, would belie this myth.

We fully empathize with clinicians' concern about the increased length of time involved in assessments such as those used by the MIDAS project. Zimmerman and Mattia state in their article:

> In the current healthcare reform zeitgeist, limits are placed on the time clinicians spend on evaluation and treatment. With managed-care companies expecting more patients to be evaluated in less time, it is logical that the frequency of missed diagnoses will increase if insufficient time is allotted to the diagnostic examination. (p. 183)[6]

Managed care companies in the United States are not alone in these expectations. In Canada's public health care system, patient throughput is the priority and quality of care is not monitored.

In addition to a comorbidity lens, we suggest viewing the results of Zimmerman's study through a lens of complexity.

Figure 5.1 illustrates the relative superiority of comprehensive assessments in identifying comorbid DSM diagnoses versus practice as usual. The

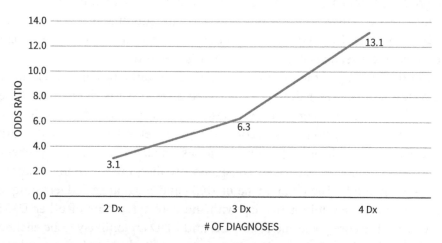

Figure 5.1 The superiority of comprehensive assessments in identifying comorbid DSM diagnoses versus practice as usual. The difference is expressed as odds ratios provided in the publication.

Adapted from Zimmerman and Mattia.[6]

difference is expressed as odds ratios provided in the publication. The graph shows that as the number of comorbid diagnoses increases, the superiority of the structured assessment also increases. In other words, the more complex the patient presentation, the less trustworthy is our typical method of unstructured assessment.

As stated previously, it is possible that some clinicians ignore the evidence that structured assessments identify more "diagnoses" by virtue of believing that such assessments are unsophisticated checklists. With respect to practice as usual, Zimmerman and co-authors support this point by stating that "it is possible that the lower comorbidity rates in the clinical sample are the result of the clinicians' deliberate underdocumentation of psychopathology" (p. 186).[6]

It is helpful at this point to have a patient perspective on the salience of the additional diagnoses identified through comprehensive structured assessments. Zimmerman and his team provided patients with information about their multiple diagnoses to gauge their wishes for treatment of these. Patients confirmed that the diagnoses related to their reasons for attending the service 50–85% of the time. They also expressed gratitude for the number of questions asked and felt more understood.[7] This finding reduces the validity of arguments that suggest structured assessments yield diagnoses that are artifacts of the method, of no interest to patients, and compromise rapport.

Beyond diagnostic considerations, the identification of comorbidity may assist in the recognition of impairment and risk of harm that transcend diagnosis. Comorbidity signals increased complexity and is associated with risk of greater psychosocial impairment. In addition, shifting from a view of our clinical task as a discrete, time-limited act to a longitudinal process, the presence of comorbidity is likely to assist the clinician in understanding treatment response and selecting alternative treatments over time.

Another finding of the MIDAS project that supports the clinical relevance of comorbidities revealed by the structured assessment is the nature of the identified disorders. For example, obsessive–compulsive disorder [OCD; practice as usual, 2.4% ($n = 12$); comprehensive method, 9.2% ($n = 46$)] and body dysmorphic disorder [BDD; practice as usual, 0% ($n = 0$); comprehensive method, 3.0% ($n = 15$)] were conspicuously absent in the cohort assessed by usual methods. The phenomena of OCD and BDD are relatively unique with comparatively minor overlap with the core symptoms of other DSM disorders. The core phenomena of OCD and BDD are unlikely to be elicited by the sweep of nonspecific interview questions. Both disorders cause high levels of distress and impairment, but the latter may be diagnosed as more common conditions such as generalized anxiety disorder or major depressive disorder or even adjustment disorder. Indeed, Zimmerman and Mattia report that when the diagnosis of BDD was fed back to patients, 70% expressed "these symptoms were among the reasons for seeking treatment" (p. 189)[6]

The unique features of OCD and BDD, combined with patients welcoming treatment for them, reduce the probability that diagnoses elicited by structured instruments are a coding artifact and irrelevant to clinical care. Zimmerman states, "Overall, 86% of the patients with depression with at least one anxiety disorder wanted their treatment to address a comorbid anxiety disorder" (p. 75).[7]

Zimmerman et al. also support findings that clinicians more frequently make a diagnosis of adjustment disorder in practice as usual, compared to the SCID, while missing conditions that require more careful and comprehensive inquiry. They found that routine assessments resulted in twice the frequency of adjustment disorders (9.6%, $n = 48$) in comparison to the comprehensively assessed group (5.0%, $n = 25$). This means that another mental disorder was misidentified as an adjustment disorder. A reason for concern is that the diagnosis of an adjustment disorder tends to lessen vigilance for disability and risk of harm. An erroneous diagnosis of adjustment disorder, therefore, could place a clinician at risk of failing to identify a client's degree of impairment and risk of harm. For instance, a study in the *American Journal of Psychiatry* reported that a diagnosis of depression was missed in 49% of cases.[8] In 68% of these missed diagnoses, the patient was instead either given a diagnosis of an adjustment disorder or identified as not having a mental disorder at all. Given the association of major depression with both intentional and unintentional death and injury, missing half the opportunities to intervene is worrisome.

Parenthetically, one can think of adjustment disorder as nonspecific and ambiguous. Isn't every mental disorder associated with diminished ability to adapt to the demands and events in life? A nonspecific diagnosis, such as adjustment disorder, is more likely to arise from diagnostic methods lacking sufficient depth and breadth of details and the nuances of a person's presentation.

It is not just uncommon disorders that are missed in cohorts assessed via usual practice methods.[6,7] Social anxiety disorder is common and was identified in only 3.2% of patients in usual practice assessments versus 28.6% in comprehensive assessments. The raw numbers matter here: 16 patients identified through unstructured assessments versus 143 in comprehensive assessments. Now imagine scaling these numbers up to a global level, or just North America alone, and consider the implications. We highlight social phobia because it is common, consistent in its presentation, and persistent, thus ensuring that untreated symptoms are present if asked about. In addition, this disorder is commonly apparent in childhood, continuing into adulthood, and relatively easy to treat. When not treated, it is associated with addiction, depression, and serious impairment. Consequently, systems have decades of opportunity to identify and effectively treat social anxiety disorder but still fail, largely due to an irrational adherence to faulty assessment methods. Overall, the MIDAS findings suggest diagnostic differences are largely due to the method of assessment rather than patients' symptoms.

Zimmerman and his team ironically voice the common concern of missing the patient's life story using structured assessments. How much more empirical evidence do we need to convince ourselves that current brief and unstructured approaches to assessment are inadequate? While other illnesses have dropped in their relative position on lists of proportional contribution to years lived with disability and disability adjusted life years, mental disorders have rapidly climbed. Our current approaches are clearly failing to reduce this burden of illness.

Another View into Diagnostic Error

Shear et al. have also investigated agreement between diagnoses made using DSM-IV SCID and practice as usual.[8] They conducted a study in western Pennsylvania including two community mental health outpatient clinics, representing urban and rural settings.

In this group's protocol, the same patient received diagnoses derived from two separate sets of clinicians. One set of clinicians made diagnoses by practice as usual and the other clinicians used a comprehensive, structured assessment in the form of the SCID and additional scales. The study compared diagnoses in 164 patients. This protocol allowed for greater confidence in judging the diagnostic discrepancies as errors because the subjects were each assessed using both approaches.

The findings are highly consistent with those of Zimmerman's group. Overall, Shear and colleagues found very poor agreement in diagnoses, with a kappa of 0.24.[8]

Shear et al. summarized the findings from singular diagnoses into six clusters they named "All bipolar disorders," "All (other) mood disorders," "All anxiety disorders," "All eating disorders," "All substances use disorders," and "All adjustment disorders." Agreement was most likely across diagnosis of mood disorders (not including the range of bipolar disorder diagnoses), with a kappa of 0.33. Adjustment disorders as a group were associated with the least agreement, with a kappa of 0.07. To appreciate these findings pragmatically, this means that the probability of diagnostic error in the mood disorder cluster was 67% and a whopping 93% in adjustment disorder diagnoses.

Figure 5.2 provides a quick overview of diagnostic agreement between clinicians using the SCID and those using practice as usual. Notice that the y axis goes lower than zero into the negative range. How can it be possible for judgments to agree less than zero? Basically, it is because the kappa statistic considers the probability that random guesses could agree. A negative kappa means that the agreement is worse than guessing.

We assert that the superiority of structured assessments over unstructured interviews is based on the method, not who is using it. In contrast, Shear et al. report, "The primary diagnosis is the one that, in the judgment of the interviewer, should be the focus of treatment" (p. 582).[8] The interviewers to whom Shear et al. refer are the clinicians performing the comprehensive assessments including the SCID. The authors, however, did not provide the determinants of the interviewer's judgment, and so we are left with questions. Was it based on the diagnosis's contribution to impairment? Asking the patient about what symptoms they most wanted assistance? The association with risk of harm or other variables? This again raises the question of how clinicians are expected to know what facet of a presentation, as coded by a diagnosis, is *primary*.

More to the point, what evidence do we have that the concept of primary diagnosis is valid. There is certainly no discussion in the DSM about the degree of certainty that a clinician can have in one diagnosis versus another. All diagnoses are equal under the nosology. To select a primary diagnosis from a

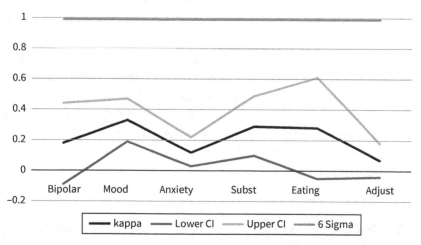

Figure 5.2 Kappa and confidence intervals plotted for each of the six categories of diagnosis defined by Shear et al.[8] Bipolar, all bipolar disorders; Mood, all mood disorders; Anxiety, all anxiety disorders; Subst, all substance use disorders; Eating, all eating disorders; Adjust, all adjustment disorders.
Based on data from Shear et al.[8]

set of diagnoses in the absence of a transparent rationale can only be guessing, which in turn requires faith or ignorance. In keeping with fully informed consent, the minimum would be to inform the patient that they meet criteria for all of x, y, and z diagnoses. The patient should then be asked which *symptoms* are the most distressing to them and informed about which diagnoses cover those symptoms so they can choose their treatment focus. The next question concerns what type of choice is being made by the patient. Are they choosing which diagnosis to treat first? Which diagnoses not to treat at all? This brings us back to the conundrum associated with complex adaptive systems. How do we rationalize an underlying assumption related to the concept of a primary diagnosis when we have absolutely no way of knowing the relative validity, if any, of DSM diagnoses? In addition, we cannot know the way in which the symptoms interact, much less the larger interaction of the syndromes coded by the symptoms.

What we do know from the evidence is that clinicians are more likely to be wrong than correct in their diagnoses. To utilize an approach that encourages clinicians to randomly select one from the list of probable diagnoses reflecting a patient's symptoms leads to an idiosyncratic deconstruction of the patient's presentation and amplifies the probability of error. This obfuscates the complexity of the presentation, tosses out the benefits provided by diagnoses as tools (e.g., alerting the clinician to complexity, range of treatment options, impairment, and risks of harm), attenuates clinical curiosity, and contributes to unwarranted certainty. To add the suggestion that one of the correctly coded diagnoses is more valid than another amplifies this unwarranted certainty severalfold.

Although our propensity to diagnostic error is concerning, it is expected when mental health is viewed through the lens of complex adaptive systems and the uncertainty inherent to them. Combined with our categorical nosology and limited diagnostic methods, errors become more likely. What is surprising, however, is the level of overconfidence in our diagnoses. Chapter 6, we illustrate the extent to which clinician confidence corresponds to objective uncertainty and clinician error.

References

1. National Academies of Sciences, Engineering, and Medicine. *Improving Diagnosis in Health Care*. National Academies Press; 2015.
2. Graber M. Diagnostic errors in medicine: A case of neglect. *Jt Comm J Qual Patient Saf.* 2005;31(2):106–113.

3. Kotwicki R, Harvey PD. Systematic study of structured diagnostic procedures in outpatient psychiatric rehabilitation: A three-year, three-cohort study of the stability of psychiatric diagnoses. *Innov Clin Neurosci.* 2013;10(5–6):14–19.
4. Martin MS, Hynes K, Hatcher S, Colman I. Diagnostic error in correctional mental health: Prevalence, causes, and consequences. *J Correct Health Care.* 2016;22(2):109–117.
5. Falissard B, Loze JY, Gasquet I, et al. Prevalence of mental disorders in French prisons for men. *BMC Psychiatry.* 2006;6:33.
6. Zimmerman M, Mattia JI. Psychiatric diagnosis in clinical practice: Is comorbidity being missed? *Compr Psychiatry.* 1999;40(3):182–191.
7. Zimmerman M. A review of 20 years of research on overdiagnosis and underdiagnosis in the Rhode Island Methods to Improve Diagnostic Assessment and Services (MIDAS) project. *Can J Psychiatry.* 2016;61(2):71–79.
8. Shear MK, Greeno C, Kang J, et al. Diagnosis of nonpsychotic patients in community clinics. *Am J Psychiatry.* 2000;157(4):581–587.

6

Confidence Versus Error

In Chapter 5, we discussed the high rates of diagnostic error in mental health care. In this chapter, we contrast this lack of accuracy with the abundant confidence that clinicians have in their assessments. Our intention is to convey two key messages. First is that this confidence is misaligned with the level of objective uncertainty inherent to our clinical assessments. Second, the degree of confidence we have in our diagnostic impressions is a remarkably poor indicator of whether we are correct. This discordance between clinician confidence and accuracy is, however, predictable; we are consistently overconfident regardless of discipline and experience levels.

Although we previously addressed uncertainty, it is necessary to clarify how it relates to clinical confidence. In the literature, uncertainty is discussed as objective or subjective. However, its opposite is usually referred to as clinician confidence instead of subjective certainty. In fact, in searching the literature, we found that it is clinician confidence that is measured and rarely certainty. Consequently, we primarily refer to subjective certainty as confidence.

Overconfidence in clinical judgment is not hubris. Most of us accept that clinical judgment is vulnerable to error, but this awareness does not assist clinicians with appreciating its frequency or recognizing which of their diagnoses are correct and which are not. Accuracy and error feel the same to us. Several forces likely reinforce our default overconfidence. First is the absence of direct and consistent feedback regarding the accuracy of our assessments throughout our careers. We are not referring to someone simply providing us verbal feedback based on their observation of an assessment. We are referring to the absence of outcome measures that an assessment was wrong or right. This is a vexing and pervasive problem in mental health that is aggravated by the delay between our assessments and final outcomes. In addition, the lack of both specificity and effectiveness of our interventions makes all outcomes ambiguous regardless of delays. The degree of difficulty in clarifying whether a clinician has made a judgment error has even conspired to reduce the probability that a clinician will experience a malpractice suit related to a mental disorder. As uncomfortable as it might be, we rarely have the benefit of litigation to facilitate calibration of our subjective confidence.

At an individual level, subjective confidence can be described as an estimate of one's own probability of error in making judgments or decisions. Most clinicians, however, neither think about nor calculate their probability of error; we simply do not think about mistakes. It requires a focused discussion of accuracy and direct questioning about confidence to elicit a clinician's confidence level. Even then, what is expressed is usually *feelings* of confidence.

In his book, *On Being Certain: Believing You Are Right Even When You're Not*, neurologist Robert Burton writes, "The feelings of knowing, correctness, conviction, and certainty aren't deliberate conclusions and conscious choices. They are mental sensations that happen to us" (p. 218).[1] Such overconfidence in our conclusions is not unique to clinicians. It appears to be a default of the human mind. This tendency for humans to exhibit overconfidence in their judgments and decisions has been referred to as the overconfidence bias.[2] The latter term alone, however, does not convey one of the more perplexing characteristics of overconfidence. It appears to be highly resistant to reduction. Indeed, overconfidence is so expected in healthy minds that low self-confidence, gross indecision, and worry about decisions are features of several mental disorders.

Our preference for confidence extends beyond our self-perception. Humans prefer the opinions and predictions of experts and authorities that portray higher levels of confidence. This is true of consultants in any domain.[3] Combining the tendency toward being overconfident in our own judgments and preferring opinions that are expressed confidently by others makes it clear that humans prefer confidence to doubt. Oddly, we are persuaded more by portrayed confidence than verifiable fact, even when facts matter. This means that clinicians exhibiting high levels of confidence in their judgments are likely to be more valued by patients, colleagues, and supervisors.

It appears that both within and outside of professional spheres, people welcome confidence as a salve for the discomfort of uncertainty. We will illustrate, however, that stupefy is a more accurate description for the numbing effect that overconfidence has on our awareness of error.

Relationship Between Clinician Confidence and Diagnostic Error

As discussed previously, the probability of a diagnostic error in mental health assessments ranges from 5% to 100%. We expect most readers will remain skeptical of this range. Even for clinicians swayed by the evidence, we tend to believe that we are the exception and that the propensity to error does not apply to *me*. Regardless of talent, brilliance, and experience, the number of unknowns in clinical practice ensures that all clinicians will make frequent errors in their judgments and decisions.

The extent to which we can mitigate the factors contributing to objective uncertainty has the potential to alter the probability of error—for instance, by performing a laboratory test to clarify if a patient's presentation relates to a drug. We cannot, however, mitigate all the factors contributing to uncertainty. For example, in the case of lab tests, we must consider the rates of false positives and false negatives as well as the integrity of the sample, equipment calibration, and the potential for human error throughout the process. Thus, there will always remain a degree of uncertainty in every judgment and decision we make. One can well imagine the difficulty in holding such uncertainty in mind at all times.

The impact of irreducible uncertainty on professional judgment greatly exceeds the triviality implied by the aphorism that *nothing is certain*. Besides, clinicians usually add, there is nothing we can do about it if the uncertainty is truly irreducible. It is the irreducibility of uncertainty, however, that makes clinician overconfidence so incongruous. We can take some action to mitigate the negative effect of unwarranted confidence on tasks such as appreciating the fallibility of history taking, actively using comprehensive differential diagnoses, and recognizing information gaps, and. It may be, however, that we cannot rely on individual clinicians to consistently reduce their unwarranted confidence because they do not subjectively experience it as unwarranted or excessive. If so, we need to consider alternative approaches to assessment and management that account for the inevitability of error and, by doing so, mitigate their impact.

Alternative Views to Diagnostic Uncertainty

Disagreements on the definition of diagnostic uncertainty are common. The article by Bhise et al. captures a common position found in the literature.[4] In a thorough review of 123 carefully selected articles, this highly experienced group of researchers from Houston, Texas, was unable to find consensus on a definition of uncertainty related to diagnosis.[4] This review led these researchers to suggest their own definition of diagnostic uncertainty. Specifically, Bhise and colleagues state, "Based on review findings, we propose that diagnostic uncertainty be defined as a 'subjective perception of an inability to provide an accurate explanation of the patient's health problem'" (p. 103).[4] The definition fails to recognize the overwhelming evidence that clinicians tend to be oblivious to the degree of objective uncertainty during and after assessing a case. The lack of subjective uncertainty is reflected in the high levels of confidence they express about their judgments.

Bhise et al. write, "Diagnostic uncertainty impedes the clinician's ability to act or think appropriately to initiate definitive treatment for the stated problem" (p. 104).[4] It also appears that these authors do not appreciate that the absence of subjective uncertainty and, by extension, the ubiquity of unwarranted confidence is a greater cause for concern, particularly from the patient perspective. Research has consistently found that when clinicians experience unwarranted confidence, they are less likely to utilize resources to assist in making an accurate diagnosis.[5]

We argue that overconfidence has the potential for doing greater harm to patients than subjective uncertainty. Unwarranted certainty increases the risk that clinicians will fail to recognize an error and, therefore, neither think about it nor take action to mitigate such a probability. Unwarranted certainty also disables the clinician from incorporating information that suggests a diagnostic error or the need to revise the differential diagnoses.

Bhise et al. also assert that "clinicians are unable to initiate definitive treatment while trying to reduce their diagnostic uncertainty through various options" (p. 105).[4] This statement reflects the common view that diagnosis is essential *before* treatment can commence, but we know that this is simply not true. First, there always remains a significant amount of irreducible uncertainty in all but a handful of diagnoses. In addition, clinicians are frequently faced with situations in which they must intervene to support life or provide comfort long before an accurate diagnosis is achieved. Therefore, this view of diagnostic uncertainty is incomplete and incompatible with the evidence in the judgment and decision-making literature.

How Much Confidence Can We Have in Our Diagnostic Accuracy?

We can think of overconfidence in several ways. At the micro level, it reflects the confidence that we experience with each of our judgments or decisions. At the macro level, it reflects the default confidence that frames all our clinical judgments. Clinicians are trained to be experts in their field. We are trained to know rather than to seriously consider what we do not know and how to move ahead accordingly. It is impossible to anticipate the degree of confidence a clinician should have with each judgment and decision they make. However, it is possible to suggest an upper limit of confidence that clinicians should have in their diagnostic accuracy.

A reasonable place to start is with the diagnostic accuracy rates revealed by existing evidence. As discussed in Chapter 5, this accuracy hovers around 50%, essentially a coin flip. Logically, the degree of confidence we have in our judgments should not exceed that figure. But it does, because logic is not our default.

How Much Confidence Do We Have?

Studies that simultaneously measure clinician confidence and assessment accuracy provide us a clear view of the degree of discordance between them. In addition to diagnosis, another common aspect of a mental health assessment prone to error is risk of harm. One such investigation was a study beginning with a naturalistic examination of clinicians' accuracy in judging patients' risks of harm within a forensic setting.[6]

The purpose of the study was to investigate the relationship between clinician accuracy and subjective confidence in predicting various risks. There are several methodological aspects of the study that make it particularly useful. Clinicians represented multiple disciplines, the numbers of patients and repeated assessments were relatively large (patients, $n = 119$; assessments, $n = 237$) for a naturalistic study, and the clinicians had access to extensive retrospective and prospective information because the average length of stay was 3 years. In addition, most patients were observed for an average of 43 weeks.

Clinicians assessed the risk of patients exhibiting four behaviors—violence, unauthorized leave, self-harm, and suicide—using a standardized instrument common to forensic mental health settings. The results indicated that clinicians were modestly better than chance in predicting patient violence, self-harm, and suicide ($r_{pb} = 0.23$; $p < .001$) and failed to perform better than chance in predicting unauthorized leave.[6] The lack of accuracy is particularly striking considering the prolonged length of stay and periods of observation.

Clinician confidence was measured by asking them to rate their level of agreement with the following statement: "I am confident in the accuracy of my assessment."[6] Overall, most clinicians rated themselves as more confident than not, with average ratings of 3.84 on a 5-point Likert scale. The authors also found a negative correlation between confidence levels and accuracy. The group of clinicians who expressed lower confidence tended to be more accurate in their assessments, particularly in predicting verbal aggression or self-harm. In contrast, the high confidence group was not more accurate on any risk. This is consistent with other studies that have found persons who rate themselves as relatively less confident exhibit better accuracy in their judgments.[3] Of note, the authors also found that confidence levels did not differ across the disciplines conducting the assessments. This is relevant because it refutes a common belief in health care that medical doctors (in this case, psychiatrists) tend to be more prone to overconfidence than those in other disciplines.

Rather than reviewing all the mental health care studies contrasting clinician confidence levels with judgment accuracy, we refer to an excellent meta-analysis of this literature published in 2015 by Miller and colleagues.[7] These authors reviewed literature from 1970 to 2011, selecting research that studied mental health clinicians from multiple disciplines, including psychiatrists but excluding primary care providers. The exclusion is notable because, internationally, the majority of mental health care is delivered by primary care. Limiting the analysis to mental health specialists may bias the cumulative accuracy of clinician judgment to be higher than if all providers of mental health care were included. This potential bias is balanced by the simultaneous collection of the confidence levels associated with the said accuracy.

The final analysis was based on 36 studies including 1,485 clinicians. The types of judgments examined represented the full range of those that clinicians must regularly make. The authors found a very small correlation of 0.15 between the confidence clinicians had in their judgments and their confirmed accuracy. The implication is that

> while counseling and other psychologists may think they are very accurate (and indeed, in most studies clinicians reported that they were quite confident in their judgments), the feeling of confidence should continue to be viewed as marginally indicative of decision-making accuracy. (p. 561)[8]

Our concern in mental health care should be clinician overconfidence, as opposed to subjective uncertainty, because of its ubiquitous and consistent influence on human judgment and because the influence suppresses prudence and corrective measures. A minority of clinicians may tend toward a lack of such confidence, and all clinicians are likely to experience it in certain circumstances. Literature that specifically addresses lack of confidence is rare—perhaps because underconfidence is as difficult to find as unicorns. The issue appears to be primarily addressed in research and opinions regarding subjective uncertainty in clinical practice. Authors in this domain express concern about the deleterious effects of clinician uncertainty on patient care, and links have been made between subjective uncertainty and therapeutic inertia.[9-11] However, these authors assume subjective uncertainty and do not measure clinician confidence to determine if clinicians are experiencing subjective uncertainty at the relevant times.

It is important to consider whether the impact of being subjectively uncertain or less confident is equal to overconfidence. Fortunately, research conducted in a variety of fields provides robust evidence to enable us to prioritize whether we should be more concerned about subjective uncertainty or overconfidence.

Evidence regarding this issue is complicated. Unwarranted confidence decreases information gathering, but gathering more information can sometimes fuel unwarranted confidence. A deeper dive into the evidence, however, consistently finds that clinician overconfidence attenuates the pursuit of information and consultation, and when additional information is pursued, its nature tends to be confirmatory of the clinician's impression, which acts to inflate overconfidence.

In research that has compared more confident clinicians with less confident clinicians, the finding has consistently been that the less confident group is more accurate in their judgments. This finding has been replicated in clinical and other domains for more than 60 years.[3,6,12,13] Tetlock's study is particularly interesting because of its real-world design and remarkably prolonged period of data collection spanning 20 years.[3] In his book describing the study and its findings, the researchers unexpectedly found that the most confident experts, despite being least accurate are more likely to be sought after for their opinions. This phenomenon has also been replicated in multiple domains.[14,15]

Miller et al. also reviewed evidence that increased years of experience may be associated with increase clinician confidence in their judgments but not increased accuracy.[8] This suggests that, unfortunately, the probability of error does not reduce as clinician experience increases. A study of clinician accuracy in diagnosing mental disorders compared three levels of experience and found that clinicians with more than 18 years of experience were not more accurate than clinical master's-level students.[16] It also found that clinicians with intermediate levels of experience between 2 and 17 years were significantly less accurate in their diagnoses than both the very experienced and novice clinicians. The lack of influence of clinical experience on accuracy has been replicated in numerous investigations for more than 50 years.[12,13,17,18] This counterintuitive finding is profoundly at odds with the celebration of clinical judgment based on experience. It is consistent, however, with the suggestion by several scholars that the absence of timely and consistent feedback about judgment accuracy and decision effectiveness precludes a critical mechanism by which clinicians might calibrate their knowledge and skills over time—a mechanism that is critical for the development of expertise in any field.

Unfortunately, studies of judgment in mental health care suffer from greater ambiguity than related studies in other areas of health care. The susceptibility to overconfidence is part of the human condition, and our colleagues in other domains, such as internal medicine, are equally susceptible to overconfidence in their judgments. By examining studies from specialties such as internal medicine, we are offered a clearer picture of the predictability and magnitude of clinician overconfidence. The study by Meyer et al. is one of the clearest on the relationship between diagnostic accuracy and clinician confidence.[13] Its methodological clarity is only surpassed by the notability of its findings.

Meyer et al. studied diagnostic accuracy in a group of internal medicine physicians selected from a cohort known to be engaged in ongoing professional development.[13] Verifiability of diagnostic accuracy was achieved by using paper cases of diagnoses with known pathophysiology and objective tests. The studied clinicians were unlikely to be less competent than the average internist because 39% of the participants worked in academic health science centers. The participating physicians also worked in 33 different states throughout the United States, representing most of the country.

The participating clinicians assessed four clinical vignettes based on validated real-world cases—two classified as easy and two as difficult. The investigators ensured that key diagnostic data w was completely available for all cases and the protocol, generally, was designed to optimize clinician probability of accuracy.

The cases were presented in a web-based format of four sequential phases: history-taking, physical examination, general diagnostic testing data, and definitive diagnostic testing. After each phase, physicians could record up to three differential diagnoses. In the language of judgment studies, they were allowed three guesses at the diagnosis after each phase. In the fourth phase, physicians were required to provide only one diagnosis. At each of the four phases, they rated their level of confidence in their diagnosis.

Confidence ratings used by Meyer and her team were clear and unambiguous. The physicians directly rated their subjective confidence on a scale that ranged from 0 to 10, with 10 being the most confidence and 0 being the least confidence.

All participants were shown the same definitive data in phase 4, regardless of what they requested. This means that if the clinician had not included the correct diagnosis in the differential or had not been considering the correct diagnosis more directly prior to phase 4, they were provided information that should have alerted them to the possibility that the diagnoses considered to that point were wrong. The overall process of working through the cases was expected to take about an hour, but physicians could do it at their leisure over several days. Figure 6.1 summarizes the results.

The simple graphs efficiently convey the primary results. The average diagnostic accuracy was 5.8% in the two "more difficult" cases and 55.3% in the two easier cases.

The degree of confidence expressed by the physician group in their rating was high relative to accuracy. The graphs clearly illustrate the relationship between accuracy and confidence. Finally, the discordances between accuracy and confidence were consistently related to unwarranted overconfidence. Physicians never underestimated their accuracy.

As part of the protocol, physicians were given opportunities to request "additional diagnostic tests, second opinions, curbside consultations, referrals, and reference materials such as electronic books"(p. 1954).[13] This feature of the study provided insight into the relevance of overconfidence to physician thinking and action in clinical settings. The higher the confidence rating,

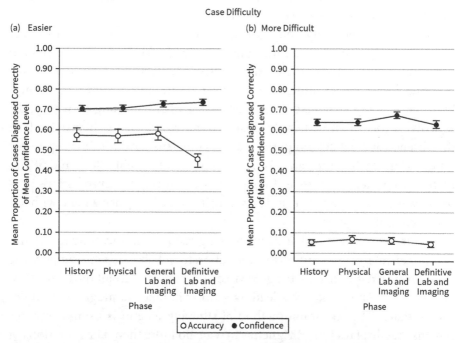

Figure 6.1 Physicians' mean diagnostic accuracy and confidence as a function of diagnostic phase and case difficulty (easier versus more difficult).

Reprinted with permission from Meyer AND, Payne VL, Meeks DW, Rao R, Singh H. Physicians' diagnostic accuracy, confidence, and resource requests: A vignette study. *INTEMED.* 2013;173(21):1952–1958, Figure 2.

the less likely the clinician was to utilize available resources. This finding demonstrates that one danger of unwarranted confidence is that clinicians stop thinking about diagnostic alternatives and therefore do not investigate them.

Meyer et al.'s findings are consistent with most reports describing the relationship between correctness and certainty in human judgment.[13] One of the pragmatic issues with unwarranted certainty demonstrated in this and other studies is that we are less likely to seek or utilize additional information to improve our probability of being correct. This is further exacerbated with increasing years of experience. Of course, why would anyone take action to reduce the chance of error in their thinking when they are already confident they are right? Confidence in our certainty shuts down curiosity and narrows our view.

Working in an academic setting also did not seem to reduce overconfidence. One might expect that clinicians in such a setting would tend toward greater circumspection and skepticism about their ability to accurately diagnose difficult cases. If clinicians are prone to overconfidence even when working in settings in which learners demonstrate the ease of error, what hope is there for those of us who do not receive such reminders?

Furthermore, the study findings suggest that neither accuracy nor respect for uncertainty improves as clinicians gain experience, and thus, we remain overconfident in our judgments and decisions throughout our careers. This immutability of overconfidence is a common finding in numerous settings but especially in domains that lack clarity on whether a judgment (e.g., diagnosis) is correct and where feedback is unavailable or rarely provided. In the absence of feedback on performance, clinicians have minimal opportunities to know when they are wrong and fewer still to calibrate thinking and methods in order to improve. To make matters worse, most professions promote values and beliefs that clinical seniority and experience equate with superior clinical judgment.

In human judgment and decision-making research, studies tend to fall into two broad categories: naturalistic and laboratory. Scholars who support the superiority of naturalistic settings have several concerns about the laboratory. For instance, Pat Croskerry, a leading scholar in medical judgment and decision, states, "The common method of studying diagnosis using computer screens that display clinical vignettes may be no more than pale imitations of what actually happens in the clinical situation" (p. 2).[19] Intuitively, this seems to make sense. An underlying assumption in this critique, however, is that the human brain is able to synthesize the entire complexity of a naturalistic setting. But we know this not to be true. Our brain takes shortcuts by virtue of the dominance of heuristics in human judgment.

In the Meyer study, if diagnostic accuracy were the only dependent variable, we would nonetheless agree with Croskerry. However, the confidence that clinicians had in their diagnoses was measured simultaneously. It is the discordance between confidence and accuracy that is important. We contend that the clinician should be able to calibrate their confidence because they are not blinded to the method of the case presentation. If a paper case does not present all the information needed, then the clinician should be aware of this and their confidence tempered accordingly.

Leaving aside its disadvantages, confidence protects us from doubt. "Doubt is an uncomfortable condition, but certainty is an absurd one." This quote, attributed to Voltaire, captures the predicament of a human faced with making a judgment in the face of uncertainty. Doubt is even more uncomfortable when both an inappropriate delay and a wrong decision can have serious consequences. It is no wonder that as health care professionals, it is much more comfortable to go about our daily work deciphering enormous complexity by ignoring uncertainty and accepting reassurance from our brain's automatic bias toward overconfidence.

We do not ascribe to the position that if we simply eradicated heuristics, cognitive biases, and other foibles, judgment and decision errors would be rare. Errors are truly inevitable regardless of clinician confidence. We need to accept that this is the reality and be compassionate toward ourselves rather than expecting the impossible.

Incorporating diagnostic processes that are designed to account for inevitable error serves both our clients and us. To this end, we next explore the trend toward transdiagnostic approaches to mental health care and how these can contribute to mitigating some of our common errors. In addition, we consider how transdiagnostic approaches can simplify diagnostic challenges while improving patient outcomes and reducing the risk of adverse events.

References

1. Burton RA. *On Being Certain: Believing You Are Right Even When You're Not.* St. Martin's Press; 2008.
2. Kahneman D, Slovic SP, Slovic P, Tversky A. *Judgment Under Uncertainty: Heuristics and Biases.* Cambridge University Press; 1982.
3. Tetlock PE. *Expert Political Judgment: How Good Is It? How Can We Know?* Second ed. Princeton University Press; 2017.

4. Bhise V, Rajan SS, Sittig DF, Morgan RO, Chaudhary P, Singh H. Defining and measuring diagnostic uncertainty in medicine: A systematic review. *J Gen Intern Med.* 2018;33(1):103–115.

5. Berner ES, Graber ML. Overconfidence as a cause of diagnostic error in medicine. *Am J Med.* 2008;121(5 Suppl):S2–S23.

6. Desmarais SL, Nicholls TL, Read JD, Brink J. Confidence and accuracy in assessments of short-term risks presented by forensic psychiatric patients. *J Forens Psychiatr Psychol.* 2010;21(1):1–22.

7. Miller FG, Cohen D, Chafouleas SM, Riley-Tillman TC, Welsh ME, Fabiano GA. A comparison of measures to screen for social, emotional, and behavioral risk. *Sch Psychol Q.* 2015;30(2):184–196.

8. Miller DJ, Spengler ES, Spengler PM. A meta-analysis of confidence and judgment accuracy in clinical decision making. *J Couns Psychol.* 2015;62(4):553–567.

9. Saposnik G, Redelmeier D, Ruff CC, Tobler PN. Cognitive biases associated with medical decisions: A systematic review. *BMC Med Inform Decis Mak.* 2016;16(1):138.

10. Saposnik G, Sempere AP, Raptis R, Prefasi D, Selchen D, Maurino J. Decision making under uncertainty, therapeutic inertia, and physicians' risk preferences in the management of multiple sclerosis (DIScUTIR MS). *BMC Neurol.* 2016;16:58.

11. Saposnik G. Applying behavioral economics and neuroeconomics to medical education and clinical care. *Can J Neurol Sci.* 2019;46(1):35–37.

12. Spengler PM, White MJ, Ægisdóttir S, et al. The Meta-Analysis of Clinical Judgment Project: Effects of experience on judgment accuracy. *The Counseling Psychologist.* 2009;37(3):350–399.

13. Meyer AND, Payne VL, Meeks DW, Rao R, Singh H. Physicians' diagnostic accuracy, confidence, and resource requests: A vignette study. *INTEMED.* 2013;173(21):1952–1958.

14. Radzevick JR, Moore DA. Competing to be certain (but wrong): Market dynamics and excessive confidence in judgment. *Manage Sci.* 201157(1):93–106.

15. Gilovich T, Griffin D, Kahneman D. *Heuristics and biases: The psychology of intuitive judgment.* Cambridge University Press; 2002.

16. Witteman CLM, van den Bercken, John H L. Intermediate effects in psychodiagnostic classification. *Eur J Psychol Assess.* 2007;23(1):56–61.

17. Kerstein RB, Radke J. Clinician accuracy when subjectively interpreting articulating paper markings. *CRANIO.* 2014;32(1):13–23.

18. Grebstein LC. Relative accuracy of actuarial prediction, experienced clinicians, and graduate students in a clinical judgment task. *J Consult Psychol.* 1963;27(2):127–132.

19. Croskerry P. Sapere aude in the diagnostic process. *Diagnosis (Berl).* 2020;7(3):165–168.

7

Mitigating Diagnostic Error Through Transdiagnostic Approaches

Independent of the validity and reliability of *Diagnostic and Statistical Manual of Mental Disorders* (DSM) diagnoses, the extent to which clinicians can confidently predicate their treatment plans on them is dependent on their accuracy. As illustrated in previous chapters, however, diagnostic accuracy is difficult to attain and impossible to verify. The problem is amplified by the confidence bias obscuring our recognition of warranted uncertainty and our own error. In addition, current approaches to mental health care, and the nosology we depend on, encourage rapid narrowing of our thinking. This leads to precariously unstable treatment plans that clinicians attempt to prop up with multiple theories and interpretations of the client's presentation. All of this perpetuates gross delays in providing people with effective interventions.

Conversely, if we accepted diagnostic uncertainty and error as a fact of clinical life, we might be more likely to develop approaches to limit their negative impact. One such strategy is to utilize assessment and treatments that are transdiagnostic. Such approaches inform management independent of where the clinician is on the continuum of diagnostic clarity or accuracy. The flexibility of transdiagnostic approaches makes them easier to apply over weeks, months, and years while clinicians amass information and explore the differential diagnosis. It is to such transdiagnostic approaches that we now turn our attention.

What Are Transdiagnostic Approaches?

What constitutes a transdiagnostic approach? Such an approach shifts our thinking from selecting one diagnosis as being correct to considering several that could all be correct. It allows us to think about treatment approaches that cut across diagnoses and include a dimensional approach. If we continue with the analogy of meteorology, a transdiagnostic approach enables us to base our actions on the possible weather rather than anchoring our actions to a singular part of the forecast. This is like checking the weather forecast when planning an outdoor activity. The forecast predicts a high of 72°F (22.2°C), a 40% change of rain, and light winds. The date is June 2, and the season is mid to late spring in a changing and unpredictable climate. You consider bringing either an umbrella or a rain jacket with a hood depending on whether you need to have both hands free. You decide to bring both to be able to respond to whatever might happen. Depending on where you are walking, you may need waterproof footwear of a certain height. The ultraviolet index is predicted to be moderate, and so you decide it does not hurt to use some sunscreen, especially if it ends up being sunny. The temperature is also expected to vary, so it is best to choose garments or layers that will prepare you for any eventuality.

Translating this into the clinical realm leads the clinician to consider what interventions best address all possibilities while minimizing a negative effect on any particular one. It is preferable to avoid the diagnostic equivalent of showing up for a group hike outside of San Francisco in March, unprepared for inclement weather. You arrive wearing breezy shorts and tank top, slathered in sunscreen, because your intuition tells you that the part of the forecast that is accurate is the 50% chance of the day being 80°F (26.6°C) and sunny, only to find yourself in a wind-driven, cold rain, ultimately being treated in hospital for hypothermia 7 hours later.

Clinically, the challenge of the weather forecast analogy is even more dramatic. Mental disorders evolve over months and years. Consequently, anchoring ourselves to one diagnosis is like deciding on a singular wardrobe based on the average temperature and rainfall for a 2-year hike through the hills and valleys of North America's national parks. This is essentially the clinical approach illustrated by research into the diagnostic and treatment histories of persons with bipolar disorder—clinicians repeatedly selecting only one aspect of the forecast and rarely revisiting the weather channel. Unlike discounting a comprehensive forecast by wearing breezy shorts on a personal hike, it is the patient who suffers the consequences of the clinician's advice. The clinician simply watches from the comfort of a climate-controlled office.

Organized approaches to undifferentiated mental/emotional states or "at-risk mental states" have increased awareness of the degree to which the evolution of symptoms is unpredictable. First episode psychosis clinics are the most obvious examples of organized approaches targeting undifferentiated mental states, even though these clinics are themselves narrowed by only accepting people with identifiable psychosis. The fact that these clinics were intended to focus on people with an early manifestation of psychotic disorders such as schizophrenia makes the unexpected findings especially potent in depicting how inaccurate are our predictions. Following patients in such clinics has revealed that not only are diagnoses uncertain but also even symptoms are not fixed over time. These fluctuations have led to unanticipated diagnostic considerations that in turn are also in constant flux. McGorry et al. summarized key findings from others—that patients initially thought to be manifesting signs and symptoms of primary psychotic disorders, such as schizophrenia, go on to manifest a range of DSM disorders outside of the psychotic spectrum, including anxiety and substance use.[1]

McGorry et al. discuss that regardless of diagnostic accuracy, "diagnosis has rather low utility for treatment decisions" and reinforces a growing appreciation that focus should include outcomes such as impaired functioning and distress (p. 135).[1] To this we add risk of harm while pointing out that this is yet another group of thoughtful authors who demonstrate how easy it is to explicitly neglect such risk. McGorry et al. ultimately make a strong case for the importance of transdiagnostic approaches to managing severe mental disorders, making it clear that experts in the field do not appreciate the potential benefit of these approaches across all perceived levels of severity.

Transdiagnostic approaches can be confused as simply giving the same assistance that is provided by a thoroughly pursued and comprehensive differential diagnosis. The important difference between a transdiagnostic approach and a differential diagnosis is that the latter does not inform the comprehensive treatment plan beyond the brief assessment phase and assumes that a correct diagnosis is inevitable. In contrast, a transdiagnostic approach assumes that several diagnoses could collectively inform ongoing assessment and management. Some transdiagnostic approaches do not even rely on discrete diagnoses and instead focus on symptoms and other phenomena. The lack of reliance on diagnoses means that transdiagnostic approaches can dramatically transform management. This directs the consideration of interventions that are applicable to the multiple conditions a client's presentation suggests, but also takes into account interventions that may worsen one or more probable diagnoses.

Some transdiagnostic approaches are more closely aligned with the specific spectrum framework of the DSM-5 but go beyond it by including conditions that are not on the same spectrum. They also align with a phenomenological approach but often incorporate the utility of diagnostic entities. For instance, a phenomenological approach might consider specific symptoms of depression in selecting treatment without considering that such symptoms are also part of bipolar disorder, alcohol-related mood disorders, or an unidentified anxiety disorder such as social phobia or body dysmorphic disorder (BDD). Management based on phenomena disconnected from diagnostic probabilities limits the scope of clinicians' perspectives, failing to inform them of potential treatments to avoid, ongoing assessment required, and treatments applicable to addiction and other disorders requiring relatively unique interventions. Diagnoses in such instances can serve as heuristic devices, cueing the consideration of potential risks associated with them.

One of the key aims of a transdiagnostic approach is to leverage time. As the degree of uncertainty increases, so does the required degree of flexibility and adaptability. Reducing an emphasis on diagnostic clarity does not preclude managing potential risks and impairments. Prioritizing the identification and mitigation of such risks buys us time to safely observe and assess the person's condition as it unfolds and, thus, enables a more comprehensive understanding of the client problems. This in turn informs comprehensive interventions that go beyond risk of harm.

As discussed previously, objective uncertainty influences both the probability of diagnostic error and the probability of error in predicting risk. Diagnostic error itself, however, can increase the risk of error in predicting risk of harm. This includes diagnostic preoccupation distracting clinicians from risk assessment or a chosen diagnosis blinding a clinician to some of the coexisting risks in a case. Consequently, we want to mitigate both the direct effects of uncertainty and diagnostic mistakes on errors of risk assessment. This is where a transdiagnostic approach would seem critical and is discussed in-depth in Chapter 8.

Limitations of Transdiagnostic Approaches

It can be said that the DSM's nosology draws perpendicularly rigid lines through horizontally woolly continua. Nonetheless, it is a useful summary of the most consistent symptoms associated with mental disorders in large populations. Viewed from this perspective, a structured comprehensive assessment based on the DSM, such as the Structured Clinical Interview for DSM (SCID), becomes a tool for a more thorough identification of symptoms. Although lengthy to administer, this cues the clinician to consider additional diagnoses along with related harms and impairment that a less complete list of symptoms often doesn't. We can consider the DSM as a useful guide or frame of reference rather than providing categorical truths.

A transdiagnostic approach is also a tool and not one of nature's rules. They have many limitations. The most obvious is in managing discrete mental disorders that require very specific interventions, particularly those that have medical causes such as symptoms of depression secondary to hypothyroidism, vitamin B_{12} deficiency, or a drug. More directly, the specifics of structured psychotherapies such as cognitive–behavioral therapy (CBT) techniques that are required for effective treatment of such disorders as severe obsessive–compulsive disorder (OCD) or severe social anxiety disorder may not be addressed by unified protocols (transdiagnostic treatment approaches) of CBT to treat emotional disorders. These limitations also pertain to disorders that are commonly comorbid with other conditions—for instance, attention deficit disorder and bipolar disorder. The problem with bipolar disorder is that a stimulant may provide transient assistance with functioning but place the patient at risk of deterioration.

However, most mental disorders currently use treatments that are nonspecific. Although a transdiagnostic approach is consistent with this current reality, we cannot abandon the pursuit of diagnostic clarification. Instead, the aim should be to ensure that we are thorough in identifying all the possible diagnoses. This enables clinicians to use all possible diagnoses as a checklist to direct attention to the diagnostic probabilities while managing the patient over time.

Interventions suggested by a transdiagnostic approach may often be a compromise. The compromise may be benign in its iatrogenic risk potential but also may not optimize treatment for any individual condition—for instance, the choice to avoid an antidepressant in a patient who presents with a probable depressive episode in an attempt to simultaneously address the probability of a bipolar affective disorder (BAD). This might be done to avoid the adverse effects of antidepressants in BAD. Specific treatments, however, are relevant to many of the medical conditions that manifest as mental disorders. In the future, when treatments become more specific to symptoms, the utility of a transdiagnostic approach may be reduced. This will require the development of both an improved nosology with conclusive validity and assessment methods capable of pointing out erroneous clinical impressions. Both are critical. Nonetheless, in health care broadly, diagnostic errors of discrete diseases with unequivocal validity are common. We need to remember that irreducible uncertainty is inherent to the complexity of the systems with which we interact. The result is inevitable errors, and the best we can do is adopt approaches that account for them.

Let's consider some existing diagnoses to illustrate the risk of completely abandoning our nosology. The failure to accurately identify diagnoses such as OCD, social phobia, and other conditions that require specific behavioral interventions is likely to limit the probability of achieving full remission. For instance, in assessing treatment response longitudinally, if all the phenomena have not been identified, then judgments of treatment response are more likely to be wrong and lead to erroneous treatment changes. In the examples of OCD, social phobia, and BDD, clinicians can often miss the opportunity to employ evidence-based psychological interventions with unique features specific to these conditions. Clinicians could also be at risk of escalating pharmacologic interventions due to their perception that a patient's condition is simply treatment refractory, rather than considering that the failure of treatment to achieve remission relates to missed diagnoses and/or related phenomena. Major depressive disorder diagnosed in the presence of an alcohol use disorder is another important and common example of such a scenario. If a clinician identifies the symptoms of depression but fails to identify the alcohol use, it is easy to conclude that failure to respond to standard antidepressant treatment is simply treatment refractory depression and then pursue more aggressive treatments with increased iatrogenic risk. These interventions are likely to include second-generation antipsychotics and other agents with side effects such as sedation. Sedation may be intensified by interaction with the alcohol and add to the risk of material harm, such as accidental injury or even respiratory depression. Failure to identify problematic alcohol use also leaves the unsuspecting clinician blind to the need to consider other risks, such as the markedly increased probability of suicide, motor vehicle accidents, child neglect or abuse, work-related issues, and the end organ effects of alcohol.

A Different Perspective on Time

Although transdiagnostic approaches may be more efficient in the long term, it may well be that weaving transdiagnostic approaches into clinical care increases the amount of time spent conducting assessments. Clinicians often say that they don't have time to engage in comprehensive assessments. We all agree that resource limits require balancing the needs of individuals with the needs of populations. The argument of insufficient time to conduct more thorough and continuous assessments, however, deserves scrutiny.

Several assumptions and beliefs are embedded within the argument. First is that patient encounters with clinicians occur over relatively brief periods. This is usually thought of in terms of the length of singular visits but obfuscates the duration over which a patient continues to require care at a system level. Second is the view that practice as usual is sufficient; therefore, the additional time required for more rigorous assessments gives a low return on investment. Stated in clinical terms, thorough structured assessments are not any better than practice as usual. Last, another common criticism is that outcomes would not change with the identification of more symptoms and more diagnoses.

We have shown that comprehensive and structured assessments are vastly superior to usual practice. One approach to examining the refrain that we do not have enough time is to consider the duration that patients remain in care for common disorders. Using this approach, we illustrate that, in mental health care, time should be measured using a calendar, not a watch.

Let us start with mood disorders and specifically one of the most diagnostically challenging due to its ambiguity, bipolar disorder. Studies describing the duration that people have had symptoms before a correct diagnosis is established provide a window into this difficulty. We highlight two studies, one published in 1994 and the other in 2013. We selected these reports in part because they are separated by almost 20 years and provide an interesting perspective on the degree to which diagnostic methods have improved over two decades. Or not.

We selected BAD because it is common and often evolves in various guises. It is easily missed or mistaken for numerous other DSM disorders. The studies included also reveal the serious consequences of delaying the diagnosis and its treatment. These consequences illustrate the effect of our reliance on discrete diagnoses and the resultant harm to people we serve.

The 1994 study by Lish et al. drew its findings from uncorroborated self-reports from members of the Depression and Bipolar Support Alliance (DBSA) in the United States.[2] These researchers directly surveyed people with lived experience of bipolar disorder. To offset the limitation associated with lack of corroboration, respondents underwent a detailed interview that gathered a wide range of information. The study provides insight into how long patients are usually in care and the multiple opportunities clinicians have to conduct thorough diagnostic assessments over time.

Lish et al. received responses from approximately 500 members of the DBSA representing 34 U.S. states. The consistency of responses coming from so many states supports the reliability of the information.

The respondents were grouped by age. The first indication of the potential impact of diagnostic error was that "Fifty percent of the respondents received no assistance for their illness for 5 years or more (p. 291)."[2] This delay in receiving care was greatest when symptoms began during childhood and adolescence."[2] Five years is likely sufficient to complete comprehensive structured assessments, should clinicians think of performing them. Only 29% of respondents reported that their diagnosis was made in less than 1 year. The fact that the delay to accurate diagnosis was measured in years is in direct contrast to the timeliness that most clinicians and clients desire. In addition, 34% of respondents reported that more than 10 years passed between their first professional contact and a correct diagnosis.

At least three or more clinicians were consulted by 48% of respondents be-fore an accurate diagnosis was made. Ten percent recalled consulting with seven or more clinicians. Clinician error is clearly not an isolated problem. The severity and clarity of respondents' symptoms were suggested by the findings that 88% of respondents reported a psychiatric hospitalization and 66% reported multiple hospitalizations. In addition, 75% of them reported an age of onset before age 25 years, and 60% were aged 19 years or younger. This is important because young age of onset, during a developmentally crit-ical period, is associated with greater severity of illness and poorer outcomes. Those reporting their first episode earlier than age 20 years had profound im-pairment in every aspect of life. Symptoms caused significantly greater school dropout (55% versus the national average of 12% at the time of publication in 1994), financial difficulties (70%), divorce/marital difficulties (73%), alcohol/drug abuse (52%), injury to self or others (46%), and minor crime (36%). These dramatic impairments illustrate the human cost of years of repeated in-adequate assessments and clinicians' obliviousness to the results of their clin-ical management.

If you are disinclined toward spending more time on assessments, then transdiagnostic approaches are even more important. The less time spent, the broader should be the differential diagnosis and the broader the scope of the transdiagnostic model. Especially important to reducing illness-related harm and impairment would be using transdiagnostic assessment models de-voted to material risks, impairment, and degree of suffering. The advantage of assessing risk of harm and impairment is that these are finite and can be con-cretely assessed. This clarifies the direction of assessment and management and informs the selection of targeted interventions. The focus on impairment and broadly defined harm would also inform less ambiguous outcome meas-ures. These in turn would serve as solid feedback to clinicians.

With the next study, we travel 20 years into the future hoping that diagnostic methods and accuracy have improved. This study eliminated confounds re-lated to the private health care system of the United States because it took place in France. The French health care system provides universal health care for both physical and mental disorders and is consistently rated as one of the world's best, based on both cost and quality. The study's subjects were exclu-sively Caucasian, reducing their chance of receiving race-based suboptimal care. There are, therefore, several reasons to expect that this study would re-flect improvements in the diagnosis of bipolar disorder relative to the 1994 American study. Or not.

Drancourt et al. surveyed 501 patients with a confirmed diagnosis of bi-polar disorder.[3] The study optimized the reliability of patient reporting by requiring a minimum of 3 months of euthymia. These subjects were recruited from university-affiliated clinics and had a higher level of education—factors usually associated with better outcomes.

Drancourt et al. identified the age at which patients first exhibited a full-blown episode of mania, hypomania, mixed or major depressive episode, as well as the age at which patients first received evidence-based pharmacotherapy (atypical antipsychotics, mood-stabilizing anticonvulsants, and lithium). The difference between the age of first episode and the age at which they first received acceptable treatment was calculated as the "duration of untreated bipolar disorder."

Unfortunately, delays were still measured in years, not days, weeks, or even months. Drancourt et al. found that those studied waited an average of almost 10 years before being treated with recognized pharmacotherapy. The authors stated, "The mean (duration of untreated bipolar disorder) was 9.6 years (SD 9.7; median 6). The median (duration of untreated bipolar disorder) for those with a hypomanic onset (14.5 years) exceeded that for depressive (13 years) and manic onset (8 years)" (p. 136).[3] Even a full-blown manic episode, arguably the only pathognomonic feature of bipolar disorder, was associated with an 8-year delay to basic treatment.

Young age of onset was again associated with a longer delay before appropriate treatment was provided. Those with an onset at 21 years or younger ($n = 240$) languished for an average of 12.5 years. Drancourt et al. found that the greater the duration of untreated bipolar disorder, the greater the likelihood of attempted suicide ($p = .0003$), reinforcing the risk of delaying effective treatment.[3]

Another dramatic finding was that even after a "cluster of contacts" with the health care system, the time to appropriate treatment was still grossly delayed. The first hospitalizations occurred more than a year after the first suicide attempts. The suicide attempts in turn occurred approximately 7 months after initiating any treatment (except the right one of course). Even in respondents with severe, overt symptoms, such as suicide attempts or requiring hospitalizations, correct treatment was delayed an additional 4.5 years.

In addition to the previously mentioned authors, for more than two decades, other authors have found similar delays in diagnosis in multiple countries. This is a travesty. However, our linear approach to diagnostic clarification likely contributes to the delay in implementing effective and safe interventions in BAD. Clinicians may either fail to appreciate the massive diagnostic ambiguity related to this condition or get stuck in a narrow range of diagnoses in which error is perpetuated by overconfidence. A transdiagnostic approach would enhance cognitive flexibility, avoiding the unwarranted anchoring on a singular diagnosis.

Anchoring, a cognitive bias, has a devastating impact when information emerges that does not fit with a clinician's preferred diagnosis. The information tends to be discounted and leads to failures to appropriately utilize it or to respond to changes in the clinical presentation. Failure to use new or corrected information is associated with poor outcomes and increased risk of adverse events. It is also consistent with the finding that being diagnosed with more than one condition is associated with worse outcomes.

Gathering more information from our clients using thorough and structured methods increases the number of mental disorders diagnosed per patient. Practitioners often assert that diagnosing more than one mental disorder in a person is a meaningless artifact of our nosology. This argument, however, does not withstand modest scrutiny. Independent of its validity in nature, several lines of evidence suggest that it is clinically important to identify all the possible diagnoses because they collectively reflect the complexity of presentations.

First, DSM diagnoses, as discussed previously, share numerous overlapping symptoms (phenomena). This makes the relative lack of comorbid diagnoses, identified in usual practice, conspicuous. The utilization of razor-thin differentials to guide management is even more conspicuous. Selecting one diagnosis from all potential diagnoses, suggested by the clinical presentation, requires ignoring the probability of multiple conditions. This is concerning. The DSM even encourages clinicians to disregard the full span of diagnoses in a patient presentation by advising the selection of one that they believe to be the best fit. This erroneous application of Occam's razor to mental disorders encourages us to ignore their complexity. This practice inadvertently increases errors in diagnosis and encourages unwarranted certainty.

In the study by Shear et al. that we reviewed in Chapter 5, the authors found evidence supporting a relationship between comorbid psychiatric diagnoses and impairment in interpersonal relationships. With respect to comorbidity and impairment, the more diagnoses the person had, the greater the impairment. The specific diagnoses were less relevant. This is a consistent finding across studies. Much remains unclear as to why there should be a relationship between comorbidity and impairment, although, as discussed previously, the impact of complexity is a likely factor. Because comorbidities are commonly missed in usual practice, the higher levels of impairment may be a result of incomplete or inappropriate treatment.[4–6]

A transdiagnostic approach that avoids the limitations of a singular diagnosis could be helpful in increasing the recognition of complexity. It could assist in reducing patient deterioration over time by pointing toward broad-based treatments. It could also lead to more accurately assessing a person's ability to function in critical life domains, independent of diagnosis, if the approach prioritized impairment. If the clinician is wrong in the nature and number of discrete diagnoses that they are considering, such a transdiagnostic approach at least facilitates a better chance of identifying impaired functioning. This potentially cues the clinician to revisit their overall impression. This would be especially true if the clinician observed that the degree and kind of impairment are misaligned with their diagnostic considerations.

We mentioned previously that time is a key ingredient baked into the development of a transdiagnostic approach. Beyond the experience of time pressures on the clinician, most of us do not think of time as an inescapable and powerful variable in diagnosis. Singh et al. nicely articulate the influence of time in identifying diagnostic errors:

> The evolution of diagnoses over time often makes it challenging to pinpoint a diagnostic error and operationalise diagnostic error definitions and measurements. The diagnostic process can also extend across multiple providers and in different locations. Moreover, there are no clear guidelines for "timely" diagnosis for majority of conditions. (p. 485)[7]

These issues add to the picture of the complexity of the diagnostic process and determining when an error has occurred. This is germane to mental disorders. The element of time is a confounding factor in the determination of diagnostic error. This relates to one of the key aims of a transdiagnostic approach to management—to mitigate the impact of such error on delaying time to effective treatment. A transdiagnostic approach can short-circuit such delays.

In Chapter 5 and elsewhere, we have been guided by the report published by the National Academies of Sciences, Engineering, and Medicine in defining diagnostic error and frameworks for mitigating their frequency and consequences. But does the Academies' definition, and the report generally, allow for transdiagnostic approaches in clinical care?

Operationalizing accuracy is difficult enough, yet the Academies' report also tackled the unenviable task of operationalizing "timely." With respect to timeliness of a diagnosis, the report clarifies its meaning as follows:

> Timeliness means that the diagnosis was not meaningfully delayed. However, the committee did not specify a time period that would reflect "timely" because this is

likely to depend on the nature of a patient's condition as well as on a realistic expectation of the duration needed to make a diagnosis (p. 85).[8]

The Academies' report seems to allow for no diagnosis to be made in the
absence of clarity, with the proviso that symptomatic management proceed
whenever reasonable. Whereas it may take weeks, months, or years to come
to an accurate diagnosis for some illnesses in other domains of medicine, this
is the norm in mental health care. The ambiguity and overlap in diagnostic
criteria, and their evolution over time, suggest the need for a longitudinal
view when moving toward diagnostic conclusions. The tendency to seek rapid
diagnoses in mental disorders unintentionally increases the probability of a
diagnostic error and delaying optimal interventions.

In contrast to our opinion that transdiagnostic approaches are a viable
solution to the problem of diagnostic error, Drancourt and colleagues suggest that prolonged delays in treatment "will only be significantly reduced by
more aggressive case finding strategies."[3] We would agree if, by case finding,
the authors were suggesting that diagnostic error is proven to be reduced by
using comprehensive and structured assessments. However, until a patient
presents with a manic episode, the DSM and the SCID will continue to lead
clinicians astray by not identifying that episodes of depression regularly pre-
cede the other features of bipolar disorder. Because of the ambiguity of mental
disorders, case finding as a singular solution is likely to be insufficient, despite
its necessity for improving the identification of all mental disorders. Case
finding is further hampered by the absence of objective methods to discon-
firm any mental disorder diagnosis. What might help is incorporating the inevitable degree of error inherent to our assessment methods and nosology by
including transdiagnostic approaches to the assessment of disability and risk
of harm. The belief that our assessments are sufficiently thorough and accurate does a disservice to our communities and clinicians.

Furthermore, the suggestion by our nosology that clinicians should make
progressively more refined distinctions between diagnoses—for instance, two
types of bipolar disorder (BDI and II)—is unlikely to help matters. Drancourt
et al. reported that "when diagnostic subtype was taken into account, the
median (duration of untreated bipolar) in BD-II cases presenting with depression was about 14 years compared with about 11 years for BD-I cases"
(p. 140).[3] These catastrophic failures, found in many studies, can be blamed
on our nosology's attempt to take an ambiguous set of diagnoses, bereft of
objective measures, and further deconstruct them into different diagnoses.
This is another way in which current nosology increases errors of judgment
by fostering *overprecision*. Overprecision can be simply thought of as a form

of overconfidence in which judgments neglect the full range of reasonable possibilities. This includes ignoring all the ways in which a judgment could be wrong. A suggested approach to overprecision is to encourage people to consider all potential conclusions in their judgments.[9]

There is consensus that most available treatments are not specific to specific diagnoses.[5,10–14] This applies to both biological and psychological treatments. Consequently, it would follow that the transdiagnostic effectiveness of medication and psychotherapy lessens the imperative of diagnostic clarity. This does not suggest we abandon the use of diagnoses but, rather, lessen our reliance on them as necessary and sufficient for appropriate treatment to proceed. The approach reduces the probability of overprecision in clinician judgments and decisions. Lack of treatment specificity supports the rationale for transdiagnostic treatment approaches pending the improvement in the validity of our nosology, diagnostic testing, and specificity of treatments. There is currently an international trend toward such approaches, suggesting a more unassuming view of our nosology, as well as a rational reduction in our certainty and confidence around singular diagnoses.

Clark et al.'s work is a thoughtful examination of the existing primary classification systems: the *International Classification of Diseases* 11th edition (ICD-11), DSM-5, and Research Domain Criteria (RDoC).[15] It is a sophisticated contemplation of limitations and completely relevant to clinicians and our long-standing approach to assessment and management. It is also a reflection of the ways in which a growing number of scholars are thinking about the utility of transdiagnostic approaches to address these limitations. Here, we utilize an excellent review that addresses the applicability of them to clinical practice. It is important that if we are going to identify concerns about the existing nosology, we must discuss potential solutions to these in the service of mental health care delivery.

We were struck by the parallel in some of Clark et al.'s comments to one of our assertions in a Chapter 1 that some cognitive biases may function like persistent illusions that defy our efforts to see past them. Similarly, Clark et al. suggest the following in their executive summary: "Despite the necessity of mental disorder categorization, we must resist the lure of reification and the illusion of distinct disorders" (p. 74).[15]

In alignment with our key premises, regarding uncertainty and inevitable errors, Clark et al. encourage clinicians, "Acknowledge the limitations of current diagnostic classification systems and seek out approaches to assessment and treatment that transcend them" (p. 74).[15] The authors go on to suggest that "clinical and research organizations" should "educate members about the limitations of current diagnostic classification systems, the use of dimensional assessments of psychopathology in clinical practice, and the value of thinking transdiagnostically when assessing and treating individuals with mental illness" (p. 74).[15] They make a clear statement about broadly incorporating such approaches to "work toward broadening the focus of your society, its journals, and its internal organization to incorporate transdiagnostic, dimensional approaches to psychopathology" (p. 74).[15]

Clark et al.'s paper considers multiple stakeholders. The suggestion to "universities and institutes" is to "take the lead in developing and disseminating transdiagnostic and dimensional approaches to preventing, assessing, and treating psychopathology" (p. 74).[15] With a gentle tone of admonishment, the authors also suggest universities and institutes "consider how your institution's organizational structure may contribute to narrow diagnostic thinking rather than broader transdiagnostic, dimensional approaches to mental illness" (p. 74).[15]

Clark et al. provide some interesting examples of studies illustrating some of the limits of diagnoses and advantages of a phenomenological approach. For instance, they report on the findings by Brittain et al. showing that diagnoses were inferior to symptom dimensions in predicting several clinically important outcomes, such as aggressive behavior, self-injury, and activities of daily living (ADLs).[16]

We suggest that one of the advantages of a transdiagnostic approach that focuses on risk of harm, functional impairment, and distress is that it transcends dimensions and diagnoses. Such an approach attends to the concrete manifestations of mental disorders that have the potential for a devastating impact. Indicators of actual harm and impaired functioning are considerably easier to operationalize, are directly observable, and are often measurable. For instance, death and injury tend to be relatively clear, as are the consequences of impaired ADLs. Similarly, in the domain of impaired functioning, a reduction in bathing lends itself to quantitative measurement. This can also be said of numerous areas of basic and instrumental ADLs.

Attempts to indirectly assess risk of harm, degree of impairment, and distress using diagnoses and formulations are unlikely to be successful. As Clark et al. note, "We currently have little understanding of how disability and distress arise in individuals with mental disorder(s), including the roles of individual symptoms, environmental factors, and other intrinsic factors not directly related to specific symptom criteria" (p. 116).[15]

The unified protocol for transdiagnostic treatment of emotional disorders illustrates this notion by emphasizing the commonalities in phenomenology, risk factors, and treatment response across a wide range of disorders.[13] The extent to which our current categorization of mental disorders is embedded within every aspect of our health care system requires an introduction of transdiagnostic approaches while continuing to carefully use our nosology. Pragmatically, we are suggesting using both. Transdiagnostic approaches need to work synergistically with existing nosology if they are to be adopted and therefore have utility—at least until we have a nosology that is valid and does not encourage overprecision.

Comorbidity Remains Important

Despite considerable alignment with our thinking regarding the limitations of our system of diagnosis, we disagree with Clark et al.'s view of comorbidity. Consequently, a further discussion of comorbidity is relevant to a perspective that integrates transdiagnostic approaches with the existing nosology. Clark et al. make the following statements: "The rampant comorbidity of current mental-disorder diagnoses is artifactual but not random" and "comorbidity is an indicator of an imperfect classification system; available steps should be taken to reduce it and clinically viable approaches sought to manage it" (p. 74).[15] In fairness to Clark and colleagues, there are aspects of the paper discussing comorbidity that make sense when considering a dimensional approach. For instance, the authors question the wisdom of subclassifying mood disorders into entities such as double depression, persistent depressive disorder, major depressive episode, and then additional distinctions made using "specifiers"—more examples of the nosology encouraging overprecision. Although it is relevant to study progressively more deconstructed elements in a research setting, the applicability at a clinical level, given the enormous rate of diagnostic error, is dubious at best. It takes clinicians an average of 10 years even to make the distinction between bipolar disorder and a range of other disorders. Many clinicians cannot even distinguish major depressive episodes from adjustment disorder, and yet they are asked to make an accurate distinction between the symptoms of persistent depressive disorder and major depressive disorder.[4-6]

Our point of disagreement with Clark et al. is with their suggestion that all disorders coded for within a single individual, during the same presentation, are an artifact of nosology.[15] As we illustrated in previous chapters, there are several disorders that clinicians in usual practice fail to identify despite the robustness of their symptomatology and patients' wishes to have the relatively discrete symptoms treated. OCD, BDD, and social anxiety disorder are examples of disorders that are missed and overlap minimally with other conditions. Similarly, the identification of substance use disorders is critical in teasing out what constellations of symptoms are secondary to the effect of the substance or appear to have a life of their own. We do not dispute that these comorbidities could result from the same underlying pathway or maladaptation of the complex adaptive systems of the brain and mind. We do not yet, however, have supporting evidence for this. It is the clinical utility of having a system that allows us to describe co-occurring "conditions" and their associated phenomena which compels us to disagree with a blanket statement that all comorbidity is simply an artifact of our nosology.

Emerging Transdiagnostic Approaches in Mental Health Care

Throughout this book, we have elucidated the inherent uncertainty and complexity of mental illness and the many challenges associated with the current system of classification. Our collective reliance on and confidence in it have led to problems. Such problems include reinforcing numerous cognitive biases, an oversimplification of mental disorders, significant treatment delays, missing important symptoms, and overconfidence in our diagnoses and subsequent management. This of course, for many, has called into question the utility of the diagnostic frame. Hence the movement toward transdiagnostic approaches to assessment and management. These approaches may be viewed as "soft" or "hard." The former uses the diagnostic framework but uses treatments that cut across these diagnoses, whereas the latter eschews diagnoses, focusing instead on the observable phenomena of mental disorders.[14] One example of the soft approach is the Hierarchical Taxonomy of Psychopathology, a classification system that is dimensional, data-driven, and uses DSM diagnoses that align with various spectra.[17] An example of the hard approach is the RDoC. This is an atheoretical framework to the classification of mental illness for research purposes. It does not use diagnostic categories and is based on observable phenomena and neurobiology. Clustering phenomena into groups that reflect common elements (linking diagnoses) and/or drivers, such as perceived threat in the case of anxiety, allows for broader and more heterogeneous approaches to both assessment and treatment.

Some of the criticisms directed at transdiagnostic approaches are that they are atheoretical, develop out of clinical experience rather than the laboratory (although the RDoC is a research taxonomy), are not well researched, and are too broad to capture symptoms that fall at dimensional extremes. Although it is in early days for these approaches to mental illness, it is important that the complexity of mental disorders and our previous ways of thinking about them are being explored. Proponents of the transdiagnostic approaches to assessment and management view them as having a wider reach, easier and more cost-effective to teach and scalable. Most of the psychological treatment approaches, including the unified protocol, rely predominantly on CBT, the most researched of the psychotherapies.[18] This is potentially problematic given the focus of CBT to primarily address cognition and its content. This may narrow the field's consideration of other useful, acceptable, and accessible approaches.

We question the criticism that transdiagnostic approaches are problematic because they are atheoretical. First, the approaches are aligned with an evidence-based approach to improving judgment and decision making by mitigating characteristics of traditional diagnostic approaches that are undeniably error-prone. In addition, they are in keeping with the nonspecific nature of existing treatments for common mental disorders. They chart a course of reducing the delay to treatment resulting from diagnostic error and overprecision. Finally, transdiagnostic approaches are a means of reconfiguring our existing nosology—doing so in a manner more consistent with a complex adaptive system theory of the brain and reducing the reliance on linear theories to explain the nonlinear properties of the human mind. In summary, rather than being atheoretical, transdiagnostic approaches are consistent with theories typically ignored by mental health. Such theories broaden our thinking to consider novel solutions that may mitigate existing deficiencies in mental health care.

Summary

In this chapter, we considered the use of transdiagnostic or phenomenological approaches to assessing and treating mental health and addictions problems. What is common to our current approaches is how narrowly they identify the range of harm and impairment that can be associated with disrupted mental health. In the following chapters, we suggest a novel transdiagnostic approach to comprehensively identifying risks of harm and impairment while accommodating for the objective uncertainty and complexity intrinsic to clinical practice.

References

1. McGorry PD, Hartmann JA, Spooner R, Nelson B. Beyond the "at risk mental state" concept: Transitioning to transdiagnostic psychiatry. *World Psychiatry.* 2018;17(2):133–142.

2. Lish JD, Dime-Meenan S, Whybrow PC, Price RA, Hirschfeld RM. The National Depressive and Manic–Depressive Association (DMDA) survey of bipolar members. *J Affect Disord.* 1994;31(4):281–294.

3. Drancourt N, Etain B, Lajnef M, et al. Duration of untreated bipolar disorder: Missed opportunities on the long road to optimal treatment. *Acta Psychiatr Scand.* 2013;127(2):136–144.

4. Zimmerman M, Mattia JI. Psychiatric diagnosis in clinical practice: Is comorbidity being missed? *Compr Psychiatry.* 1999;40(3):182–191.

5. Zimmerman M. A review of 20 years of research on overdiagnosis and underdiagnosis in the Rhode Island Methods to Improve Diagnostic Assessment and Services (MIDAS) project. *Can J Psychiatry.* 2016;61(2):71–79.

6. Shear MK, Greeno C, Kang J, et al. Diagnosis of nonpsychotic patients in community clinics. *Am J Psychiatry.* 2000;157(4):581–587.

7. Singh H, Schiff GD, Graber ML, Onakpoya I, Thompson MJ. The global burden of diagnostic errors in primary care. *BMJ Qual Saf.* 2017;26(6):484–494.

8. National Academies of Sciences, Engineering, and Medicine 2015. *Improving Diagnosis in Health Care.* Washington, DC: The National Academies Press. https://doi.org/10.17226/21794.

9. Haran U, Moore DA, Morewedge CK. A simple remedy for overprecision in judgment. *Judgm Decis Mak.* 2010;5(7):467–476.

10. Maher AR, Theodore G. Summary of the comparative effectiveness review on off-label use of atypical antipsychotics. *J Manag Care Pharm.* 2012;18(5 Suppl B):S1–S20.

11. Canadian Pharmacists Association. *Compendium of Therapeutic Choices 2019.* Canadian Pharmacists Association; 2019.

12. Brunton LL, Hilal-Dandan R, Knollmann BC. *Goodman and Gilman's The Therapeutic Basis of Therapeutics.* 13th ed. McGraw-Hill; 2018.

13. Barlow DH, Farchione TJ, Bullis JR, et al. The unified protocol for transdiagnostic treatment of emotional disorders compared with diagnosis-specific protocols for anxiety disorders: A randomized clinical trial. *JAMA Psychiatry.* 2017;74(9):875–884.

14. Newby JM, McKinnon A, Kuyken W, Gilbody S, Dalgleish T. Systematic review and meta-analysis of transdiagnostic psychological treatments for anxiety and depressive disorders in adulthood. *Clin Psychol Rev.* 2015;40:91–110.

15. Clark LA, Cuthbert B, Lewis-Fernandez R, Narrow WE, Reed GM. Three approaches to understanding and classifying mental disorder: ICD-11, DSM-5, and the National Institute of Mental Health's Research Domain Criteria (RDoC). *Psychol Sci Public Interest.* 2017;18(2):72–145.

16. Brittain PJ, Lobo SE, Rucker J, et al. Harnessing clinical psychiatric data with an electronic assessment tool (OPCRIT+): The utility of symptom dimensions. *PLoS One.* 2013;8(3):e58790.

17. Kotov R, Krueger RF, Watson D, et al. The Hierarchical Taxonomy of Psychopathology (HiTOP): A dimensional alternative to traditional nosologies. *J Abnorm Psychol.* 2017;126(4):454–477.

18. Wilamowska ZA, Thompson-Hollands J, Fairholme CP, Ellard KK, Farchione TJ, Barlow DH. Conceptual background, development, and preliminary data from the unified protocol for transdiagnostic treatment of emotional disorders. *Depress Anxiety.* 2010;27(10):882–890.

8

Priorities in Risk Assessment

In Chapter 7, we explored transdiagnostic approaches to patient assessment and how they may help mitigate the negative consequences of diagnostic limitations. We now begin to address the importance of augmenting the diagnostic assessment of mental disorders with a transdiagnostic approach to comprehensively identify risk of harm and functional impairments. This does not eliminate the need for diagnostic assessment but, rather, prioritizes potential harm and impairments independent of *knowing* a diagnosis. The intention is to uncouple thinking about risks and impairments from the diagnostic framework and, therefore, reduce the negative impact of diagnostic errors on identifying potential harm. To thoroughly address risk of harm, such an approach also needs to identify a person's functional impairments, commonly referred to as disability. In addition, attention needs to be drawn to signs and symptoms of distress that are most related to potential harm.

In this chapter, we introduce the vital risks that such an approach should incorporate using evidence to support their inclusion. In Chapter 9, we describe the approach in its entirety, integrating relevant functional impairments and critical symptoms.

The evidence for the risks we include is drawn from population-level data. Statistics and large numbers, however, are not compelling and tend to be ignored in decision making in clinical practice.[1-7] This phenomenon is often captured by the meme attributed to Stalin: "The death of one man is a tragedy. The death of millions is a statistic." Consequently, cases will be combined with statistics in an attempt to, ironically, bring the enumeration of death and injury to life.

Is Risk Identification Sufficiently Prioritized?

In our thinking about the potentially ruinous sequela of mental disorders, we have wondered whether the word "risk" is sufficiently alarming to clinicians. We have chosen to follow convention and use the term but wanted to share our doubts about it. First, *risk* has become somewhat cleansed of the unpleasant nature of the material harm that patients and those around them experience. Risk, as a concept, often refers to probabilities that are adequately predictive of events in populations but inadequate in predicting what an individual will experience. So, when we think in terms of risk, we may overestimate the ability of a probability to predict whether an individual client will experience harm. Risk is also a nonspecific term with many associations that may contribute to its euphemistic use and lack of emotional charge for clinicians. One of the conceptual pillars of the proposed approach is that clinicians make judgments and decisions primarily about individuals and in close partnership with them. When harm does occur, the therapeutic connection and clinician accountability have salience that probabilities and other numbers do not. In contrast, there is nothing intimate or personal about the term risk. We believe that a term such as *harm* is more evocative and less ambiguous in representing what we are attempting to prevent.

Currently, the diagnostic aspect of mental health assessment overshadows the identification of potential harm. Risk assessment is rhetorically emphasized, but evidence of its prioritization is difficult to find. A PubMed search revealed 3.5 times more articles on diagnosis than risk assessment and 14 times the number related to harm. We have a comprehensive, regularly revised, manual focused on diagnoses but have not put the same degree of effort into risk identification or assessment. Unfortunately, the *Diagnostic and Statistical Manual of Mental Disorders* (DSM) is conspicuously demure in facilitating a clinician's attention to risk of harm and so cannot be relied on for this purpose.

The relatively low emphasis on risk identification is also reflected in the clinical time devoted to its management in professional training and continuing professional development. Most centers that train psychiatrists, psychologists, social workers, and other clinicians spend more time fostering formulation skills and indoctrinating recruits into causal formulations. We have no equivalent conceptual model to reliably facilitate broad risk identification and the assessment of impairments. We are more likely to hear from our peers that risk assessment is difficult and fraught with error than to hear that diagnostic or causal formulations are unreliable. Clear and consistent risk assessments are difficult to find across the spectrum from community settings to locked psychiatric intensive care units. Only our forensic colleagues are likely to engage in structured or consistent risk assessments, and even then, consensus on an approach is lacking and their accuracy does not inspire confidence. The most consistent approach to risk assessment in North America and Europe is to defer the task to others by sending clients to an emergency department.

Few of our clinical practice guidelines and best practice recommendations include attention to risk of harm associated with mental disorders.[8] The data on suicide rates alone tell the real story about risk by reflecting our failure to reduce death by this method. And yet, although we lament this, we still do not prioritize risk and train clinicians in its comprehensive assessment.

While the probability of suicide is most associated with symptoms of depression, it is also associated with numerous other mental disorders.[9] Similarly, other than death by unintentional overdose related to substance use disorders, most DSM diagnoses are not associated with their own specific or unique risks of harm. Thus, it would make sense to use a transdiagnostic or phenomenological approach for identifying such.

In most U.S. states and other countries, physicians are consistently required to enter a diagnosis for a hospital admission to proceed. They are not, however, required to enter the risk of harm or degree of impairment with the same consistency. This includes admissions to mental health units. The irony is that the hospitalization of a person due to a mental disorder is rarely, if ever, because of a diagnosis or access to procedures that are unavailable in the community. It is, almost exclusively, related to issues of safety and the need for continuous monitoring in hospital while treatment is provided. It is the risk and impairment that determine urgency and hospitalization in mental disorders, not the diagnosis.

Why Prioritize Risk and Impairment?

One goal of identifying any illness is to prevent or reduce its negative impact. The merciless escalation of mental disorders' contribution to mortality and disability in North America, and throughout the world, suggests that our current approaches are inadequate. On a population scale, clinicians are positioned to collectively reduce this impact one person at a time. This would require shifting our focus from diagnosis and causal formulations to identifying risks of harm and impairment. Using recognized measures, evidence of our collective success would be reflected in decreasing the proportion of years of life lost and years lived with disability due to mental disorders. Suffering and quality of life are inextricably tied to mortality and disability. The lessening of distress and improvement of quality of life are important indicators of success. These measures are not, however, consistently reported by governments and health systems in a manner that makes them easily available to gauge the success of various approaches.

Mortality Associated with Mental Disorders

A relatively recent meta-analysis provides a solid accounting of the contribution of mental disorders to mortality.[9] However, it is interesting to note the authors' expression of a common and perplexing conceptualization of harm relating to these conditions. The authors write, "The link between mental disorders and mortality is complicated because most people with mental disorders do not die of their condition; rather, they die of heart disease and other chronic diseases, infections, suicide, and other causes."[9] The perplexing aspect of this statement is the authors' suggestion that suicide is not considered a death caused by mental disorders, though we are aware that suicide is frequently referred to in this manner. If thoughts and emotions that compel a person to intentionally end their life are common symptoms of mental disorders, then the natural extension into actions resulting in death must be viewed as a consequence of them. Discourse that suggests a disconnection between death by suicide and mental disorders perpetuates the erroneous view that they are relatively benign illnesses that do not have mechanisms that directly relate to death. Although it remains unknown if death by suicide has a neurophysiological pathway in mental disorders, we can at least assert that such death is associated with a common set of emotions, urges, thoughts, and behaviors that represent a common psychopathological pathway. To emphasize the impact of mental disorders on potential life years lost, Walker and colleagues found that the difference between "natural" (e.g., heart disease) and "unnatural" (e.g., suicide) causes of death was higher for "unnatural" causes, with a median of 21.6 versus 9.6 years lost, respectively.[9] Those with mental disorders die younger from suicide and unintentional injury than other medical illnesses that shorten lives. This begs the question of when we are speaking about an illness, mental or otherwise, and its outcomes, what makes one outcome natural and another unnatural?

Walker and colleagues also discuss some of the probable mechanisms by which mental disorders come to be associated with chronic medical conditions and earlier death. They state, "People with mental disorders have high rates of adverse health behaviors, including tobacco smoking, substance use, physical inactivity, and poor diet. In turn, these behaviors contribute to the high rates of chronic medical conditions among people with mental disorders."[9] From our perspective and reflected in our conceptualization of the interactions between risk of harm and impaired functioning in the approach we propose, it is the impact of mental disorders on basic and instrumental activities of daily living that is mostly responsible for the higher rates of medical illness and their complications. This is an important source of unintentional risk to self from behaviors that increase susceptibility to chronic medical conditions and compromise the afflicted person's ability to manage these health needs. This supports the importance of identifying and addressing impaired functioning as part of comprehensive risk identification strategies. We who work in mental health do not focus on identifying and responding to impaired functioning at a level commensurate with its devastating effect on physical and mental health, its impact on autonomy and quality of life, and its contribution to disability. In contrast, there are consistent protocols for stroke rehabilitation, as there are for numerous other diseases. It is little wonder that mental disorders account for the greatest number of years lived with disability worldwide.

Current Approaches to Risk and Suicide Assessment

There are usually large gaps between guidelines or recommendations and the extent to which clinicians apply these at the point of care. It seems that our current approaches to reducing suicide and other harm are failing. Consequently, we have decided to forgo a review of available guidelines and illustrate examples of actual practice described in the literature.

Given that most mental disorders begin early in life and that suicide is a dominant contributor to death in youth, we selected a representative study related to risk assessment in this population. Investigators in the United Kingdom conducted an in-depth qualitative study involving 28 primary care physicians.[10] The clinicians noted that their training in youth suicide did not prepare them to conduct such risk assessments in practice and expressed a lack of certainty in their knowledge. Although this indicated they had insight, several other findings suggested that many clinicians were oblivious to what they did not know. For instance, the respondents expressed an inability "to distinguish between signs indicating imminent suicide risk from behavioural and affective changes that form part of normal adolescence."[10] The apparent failure to appreciate that thoughts of suicide are not a part of normal adolescence was reflected throughout the findings. This includes a worrisome trend among these physicians to categorize suicide attempts, self-harm, and expressed thoughts and feelings of suicide as "truly suicidal behaviour," a "cry for help," or normal adolescence. It is surprising how easily and consistently pedestrian concepts reflecting both stigma and lay epistemology were expressed by these health care providers. It was clear that respondents were struggling in their attempts to assess suicide risk. It was concerning that some of the youth that physicians believed were expressing "a cry for help" (a lay epistemology bias) were not provided meaningful interventions to reduce their risk because this "cry" was viewed as a very low priority. The authors state, "Rationalising self-harm as attention-seeking behaviour has been previously endorsed by health professionals, including GPs [general practitioners]" as well as those who are focused or specialized in mental health.[10]

Of greatest concern was the finding that physicians believed that people who die by suicide do not divulge their thoughts or ideas. By extension, patients who do reveal thoughts of suicide are not going to end their lives. We remind readers that this study was published in 2016, not 1916, and that respondents in this study are the core of one of the world's best health care systems. Moreover, the United Kingdom is commonly utilized by other countries as a source of best practice in mental health care. The following quote provided by the authors captures the respondents' disconcerting beliefs: "If they're going to do it, they're going to do it."[10]

Unfortunately, this common myth among the public manifests as another bias among many clinicians across numerous disciplines, including social work, psychology, and medicine. The persistence of the idea that people don't reveal the symptomatic thoughts and feelings of suicide is in direct contrast to the evidence that almost half of people with confirmed suicide deaths had contact with primary care within 1 month of death and an even higher proportion had contact with any health care service.[11-13]

With respect to the nature of the interventions commonly provided to those expressing suicidal ideation, respondents in Michail and Tait's study regularly suggested that their patients "reach out to friends and family for help."[10] This is a common feature of safety plans. In addition to being common, it is ineffective, if unwavering suicide rates are any indication. The persistence of this uninspired feature found in most safety plans is problematic and reflects (1) a lack of recognition that the health care provider is being confronted with an acute and catastrophic illness and (2) an absurd expectation that a person's social connections are capable of managing the problem that clinicians cannot.

Unfortunately, when the studied clinicians did recognize a need for care, they reported frequent barriers to accessing assistance and support from mental health specialists, often being told the cases were not high risk. This problem, ubiquitous worldwide, speaks to the importance of providing all clinicians, including those involved in primary care, with approaches to risk of harm that they can reliably utilize themselves.

To reiterate, studies suggest that 40–50% of those who die by suicide see a clinician in the prior month. Unfortunately, even when patients present with features of depression, clinicians are unlikely to inquire about suicide, and this is influenced by their diagnostic considerations.[14] If we were improving the effectiveness of our assessments and interventions, we would expect to find the proportion of suicide deaths in recently assessed patients decreasing. Although such evidence is difficult to find, research into the risk of death by suicide following discharge from a psychiatric hospitalization is readily available. The excellent population data collected in Denmark allowed a team of researchers to study 21,169 confirmed suicides over a 17-year period.[15] The peak risk of suicide after discharge was found to be within the first week and highest for shorter admissions. These findings corroborate that current risk assessments and interventions, intended to reduce the risk of suicide upon hospital discharge, have room for improvement.

Last, the study by Michail and Tait reinforces the fact that our assessments are usually subjective. The authors reported that "very often assessment of risk . . . is based on clinical judgment or 'gut feeling.'"[10] In the absence of clearly articulated best practices or training, and a lack of ability to accurately predict the likelihood of an adverse outcome, primary care providers are left to depend on their gut. It is unlikely that these same physicians and their regulating bodies would ever accept that an electrocardiogram is unnecessary if a clinician's gut assured them that a patient's heart was fine. The trust in intuition also reminds us of the general resistance among clinicians to structured mental health assessments in improving their accuracy: "The majority of GPs reported serious concerns about the usefulness and acceptability of such a tool and its potential impact on the dynamics of a consultation."[10] This is a curious finding given these physicians had already expressed difficulty with establishing rapport in this cohort of patients, in the absence of tools. It is also notable that concerns about rapport are rarely raised regarding investigations commonly used to assess other risks. For instance, colonoscopies and cystoscopies as part of identifying possible cancer. Ultimately, the relationship between provider and patient is less important than safety. Another concern expressed was that a validated instrument would make more errors. Presumably, the clinicians meant more errors than the "gut feelings" they were using and the very same gut that they feared was insufficiently trained. As clinicians, we have been, as discussed previously, socialized to trust our subjective assessments. Fortunately, in this study the respondents expressed openness to tools that would guide decision making and risk assessment.

Risk Increases with Comorbidity

It is well known that meeting criteria for more than one mental disorder and/ or substance use disorder is associated with increased risk of adverse events.

Comorbid alcohol use disorder is a robust example. It amplifies the probability of death by suicide severalfold. It has also been shown that perpetrators of homicide have high rates of mental disorders and comorbid substance use. These are but two examples that reinforce the contribution of comorbidity to harm.

To elaborate, a study of Austrian homicides revealed the following diagnoses in conjunction with substance use in perpetrators that were assessed as having schizophrenia: major depressive episode, manic episode or delusional disorder, mental retardation, personality disorder, substance-induced psychotic disorders, dementia, and mental disorder/delirium due to general medical condition.[16]

Schanda et al. state, "The fact that substance use may lead to illness decompensation and violence points to the special importance of the rates of recent comorbid substance abuse/dependence for our study."[16] This emphasizes the necessity of identifying comorbidities and appropriately managing them rather than missing them, ignoring them, viewing them as secondary, or assuming that managing the other mental disorder is sufficient.

From the perspective of risk, in this case, the *comorbid* substance use should be the priority. In support of the critical nature of comorbid conditions to risk, at least one study found that alcohol use disorder increases the risk of death by suicide regardless of the presence of other diagnosed psychiatric disorders.[17] This study reinforces the importance of prioritizing risk identification independent of what diagnoses the clinician has made and which one they consider primary.

Accuracy of Risk Assessment

Errors in assessment are not limited to diagnoses. Our ability to predict harm is also poor. Even in a context optimized for accurate risk prediction, those experienced in its assessment are unable to overcome the fallibility of current approaches. An example of this is in forensic inpatient units. Despite the high base rate of events in this setting and the opportunity for clinicians to calibrate their judgment, the ability to predict adverse events is inadequate.[18] This suggests that clinicians working in general settings would be even less accurate in their risk assessments.

Regardless of setting, all clinicians rely on rudimentary assessment methods that are intrinsically fallible. Most risk assessment tools attempt to linearly predict the probability of an event based on several pieces of information. They do not consider the fluctuating nature of mental disorders and the nonlinearity of complex adaptive systems.[19] Attempts to predict the future state of a complex adaptive system are notoriously inaccurate. This is the case even in meteorology, with forecasts that are based on millions of pieces of information, that are updated every hour, and that are processed using a bank of supercomputers that have a combined processing power of 8.4 petaflops.[20] Meteorologists, nonetheless, acknowledge that they cannot predict accurately beyond a few days, and even then, there are localized variations within forecast regions. They accept that beyond a few days, their probability of error rises exponentially. This probability of error is incorporated into the National Weather Service weather warnings so that people can make plans and take steps to mitigate damage should the prediction be correct. Indeed, their mission is to "provide weather, water, and climate data, forecasts and warnings for the protection of life and property and enhancement of the national economy."[21] In mental health, clinicians are dealing with similar levels of complexity. Our assessment methods, however, do not involve sophisticated data collection and processing systems, and they do not reflect the degree of complexity in our domain. To make matters worse, clinicians are trained to grossly overestimate their ability to accurately assess the risk of harm in individual patients and do not appreciate their susceptibility to error in the way meteorologists do.

Reminiscent of the categorical nature of nosology, assessing the risk of material harm tends to use a categorical approach. Most risk assessments involve a process whereby clinicians make a prediction about the probability of a future event categorized into low, medium, and high. The approach we propose discourages the overprecision in judgment this breeds. It aims to identify all the potential risks of harm with which a client presents. It does not rank order the likelihood of identified risks into low, medium, and high because of evidence that doing so consistently fails to predict suicide and violence.[11,14,22–26] In the same way that a categorical nosology contributes to diagnostic error, delineating risk into low, medium, and high probability contributes to multiple errors, including the failure to identify the full set of risks associated with a client's presentation and inadequate management of risks deemed to be of low priority. Clinicians base their decisions almost exclusively on risks they have judged as highly likely but fail to mitigate risks in the lower categories.

Consequently, an approach to addressing risk must abate the inevitability of error in predicting harm to, or by, the individual we are assessing. The focus is shifted to risk identification for the purpose of implementing strategies to prevent or mitigate related adverse events. This is regardless of whether intuition tells us to rank order the probabilities as low, medium, or high. Risks that are judged to be medium or low may underestimate the probability of harm and therefore can preclude focused interventions to mitigate them. Instead, in the proposed approach, risks are identified simply as present or absent. For instance, the identification that a person's symptoms and presentation suggest a risk of death by suicide (suicide risk is present) does not require that the clinician go on to guess at the probability of suicide within a particular time frame. An approach that focuses on the presence or absence of a risk aligns more accurately with the clinician's task of preventing harm at an individual level.

This is in contrast to interventions that are developed at a population level, where probabilities are clear. An individual experiences events in a binary manner, not as a population does in the form of a probability. A person cannot be 20% dead within the next 2 weeks regardless of their unfortunate membership in a population wherein 20% of all members will be dead within this period. Instead, the individual will either be dead or alive within that time frame. What is important is that we reduce the risk of death by suicide in every person presenting with the risk.

It is, in our opinion, of value that the approach we propose is not diagnostically focused and does not stratify risk. In this approach, risk identification and mitigation are viewed as primary and other aspects of assessment and management as secondary. We suggest a focus on identifying the full range of risks with which a patient presents and then assessing each thoroughly, not with the aim of risk stratification but, rather, to inform the development of interventions to prevent harm and death until full symptom remission is achieved. Before discussing the list of vital risks we have selected, we must first address the issue of intentional versus unintentional risk of harm.

Intentional Versus Unintentional Harm

Current clinical focus is almost exclusively on the risk of *intentional* harm. This ignores the full range of risks and impairments seen in mental disorders and the prominence of unintentional harm in population health data. *Unintentional* is a category of death and injury used by the National Center for Injury Prevention and Control, Centers for Disease Control and Prevention, in the United States. Therefore, the categories of intended and unintended harm have been incorporated into our proposed approach. The prevalence of unintended harm is massive. For instance, the number of nonfatal, unintentional injuries presenting to emergency departments in the United States in 2018 was 25,908,331.[27] If we are not explicit about unintentional harm, mental health clinicians and researchers will not think to address it.

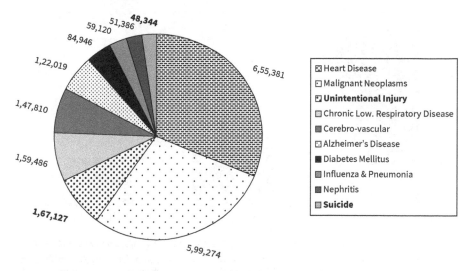

Figure 8.1 Ten leading causes of death in the United States in 2018 across all ages, races, and sexes.

Adapted from Centers for Disease Control and Prevention, National Center for Injury Prevention and Control. 10 leading causes of death, United States 2018, all races, both sexes. https://webappa.cdc.gov/cgi-bin/broker.exe.

Due to the meager categories specific to mental health in population data, however, attempts to clarify associations between these disorders and the population prevalence of unintentional harm are challenging. Nonetheless, researchers have been able to amass findings illustrating an undeniable association between mental disorders and unintentional harm.[28--33]

The fatalities from unintentional injury are a fraction of total annual injuries, but the number is still alarming. Every week, more than 3,200 Americans died from unintentional injury in 2018. Figure 8.1 shows that unintentional injury is the third leading cause of death and that suicide, mental health's dominant concern, is 10th in the United States.[34] Poisoning, of which a proportion is likely related to addiction and mental disorders, accounts for the leading cause of unintentional death at 37.3% (62,399 deaths).

The contribution of unintentional injury to death is especially dramatic for those aged 1–44 years, for whom it is the leading cause, accounting for 61,977 U.S. deaths in 2018.[34] Death by unintentional poisoning within this age group is especially high. For instance, it accounted for 66.1% of unintentional deaths in the 35- to 44-year-old age group. In addition, unintentional injury is by far the leading cause of death in the age range of 15–34 years, which covers the age of onset for most mental disorders and addiction. Figure 8.2 shows the top three causes of death in this age group.

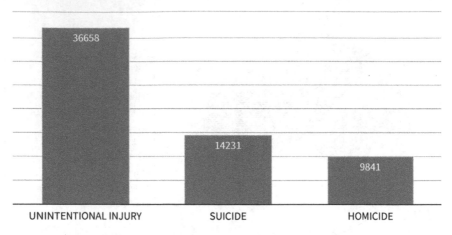

Figure 8.2 Top three causes of death in the age group 15–34 years, all sexes and races.
Adapted from Centers for Disease Control and Prevention, National Center for Injury Prevention and Control. 10 leading causes of death, United States 2018, all races, both sexes. https://webappa.cdc.gov/cgi-bin/broker.exe.

A more robust view on the impact of unintentional injury is the number of people with nonfatal injuries and poisonings who present for medical attention across the life span. This number was approximately 39.5 million in the United States in 2014.[35] These injuries often require several visits to physician offices, and in the United States in 2016, they accounted for 72.6 million visits.[35]

Summary

In this chapter, we discussed key issues that need to be considered in developing an approach to comprehensive risk identification. These include its prioritization, the range of contributors to mortality, the influence of comorbidity, and current approaches to risk assessment and their accuracy. We also highlighted the importance of incorporating unintentional forms of injury and death into risk assessment. In Chapter 9, we detail the rationale and evidence for the set of risks considered to be vital for such an approach.

References

1. Slovic P. "If I look at the mass I will never act": Psychic numbing and genocide. *Judg Decis Making.* 2007;2(2):79–95.

2. Slovic P. 41st Annual North American Meeting of the Society for Medical Decision Making; October 21, 2019; Portland, Oregon Keynote Address The More Who Die, the Less We Care: Confronting the Deadly Arithmetic of Compassion. *Med Decis Making.* 2020;40(4):407–415.

3. Västfjäll D, Slovic P, Burns WJ, et al. The arithmetic of emotion: Integration of incidental and integral affect in judgments and decisions. *Front Psychol.* 2016;7:325.

4. Västfjäll D, Slovic P, Mayorga M, Peters E. Compassion fade: Affect and charity are greatest for a single child in need. *PLoS One.* 2014;9(6):e100115.

5. Peters E, Dieckmann NF, Västfjäll D, Mertz CK, Slovic P, Hibbard JH. Bringing meaning to numbers: The impact of evaluative categories on decisions. *J Exp Psychol Appl.* 2009;15(3):213–227.

6. Peters E, Slovic P, Hibbard JH, Tusler M. Why worry? Worry, risk perceptions, and willingness to act to reduce medical errors. *Health Psychol.* 2006;25(2):144–152.

7. Slovic P, Peters E, Finucane ML, Macgregor DG. Affect, risk, and decision making. *Health Psychol.* 2005;24(4S):S35–S40.

8. Royal Australian and New Zealand College of Psychiatrists Clinical Practice Guidelines Team for Deliberate Self-Harm. Australian and New Zealand clinical practice guidelines for the management of adult deliberate self-harm. *Aust N Z J Psychiatry.* 2004;38(11–12):868–884.

9. Walker ER, McGee RE, Druss BG. Mortality in mental disorders and global disease burden implications: A systematic review and meta-analysis. *JAMA Psychiatry.* 2015;72(4):334–341.

10. Michail M, Tait L. Exploring general practitioners' views and experiences on suicide risk assessment and management of young people in primary care: A qualitative study in the UK. *BMJ Open.* 2016;6(1):e009654.

11. Shah R, Eynan R, Heisel MJ, Eden D, Jhirad R, Links PS. Confidential survey into southwestern Ontario suicide: Implication for primary care practice. *Prim Care Companion CNS Disord.* 2018;20(2):17m–2217. doi:10.4088/PCC.17m02217.

12. Luoma JB, Martin CE, Pearson JL. Contact with mental health and primary care providers before suicide: A review of the evidence. *Am J Psychiatry.* 2002;159(6):909–916.

13. Ahmedani BK, Simon GE, Stewart C, et al. Health care contacts in the year before suicide death. *J Gen Intern Med.* 2014;29(6):870–877.

14. Feldman MD, Franks P, Duberstein PR, Vannoy S, Epstein R, Kravitz RL. Let's not talk about it: Suicide inquiry in primary care. *Ann Fam Med.* 2007;5(5):412–418.

15. Qin P, Nordentoft M. Suicide risk in relation to psychiatric hospitalization: Evidence based on longitudinal registers. *Arch Gen Psychiatry.* 2005;62(4):427–432.

16. Schanda H, Knecht G, Schreinzer D, Stompe T, Ortwein-Swoboda G, Waldhoer T. Homicide and major mental disorders: A 25-year study. *Acta Psychiatr Scand.* 2004;110(2):98–107.

17. Flensborg-Madsen T, Knop J, Mortensen EL, Becker U, Sher L, Grønbaek M. Alcohol use disorders increase the risk of completed suicide—irrespective of other psychiatric disorders: A longitudinal cohort study. *Psychiatry Res.* 2009;167(1–2):123–130.

18. Desmarais SL, Nicholls TL, Read JD, Brink J. Confidence and accuracy in assessments of short-term risks presented by forensic psychiatric patients. *J Forens Psychiatry Psychol.* 2010;21(1):1–22.

19. Glancy GD, Chaimowitz G. The clinical use of risk assessment. *Can J Psychiatry.* 2005;50(1):12–17.

20. National Weather Service, National Oceanic and Atmospheric Administration. About supercomputers. https://www.weather.gov/about/supercomputers. Accessed August 29, 2020.

21. National Weather Service. The National Weather Service (NWS). https://www.weather.gov/about. Accessed August 29, 2020.

22. Buchanan A. Violence risk assessment in clinical settings: Being sure about being sure. *Behav Sci Law.* 2013;31(1):74–80.

23. Cahill S, Rakow T. Assessing risk and prioritizing referral for self-harm: When and why is my judgement different from yours? *Clin Psychol Psychother.* 2012;19(5):399–410.

24. Ryan C, Nielssen O, Paton M, Large M. Clinical decisions in psychiatry should not be based on risk assessment. *Australas Psychiatry.* 2010;18(5):398–403.

25. Garbrick L, Levitt MA, Barrett M, Graham L. Agreement between emergency physicians and psychiatrists regarding admission decisions. *Acad Emerg Med.* 1996;3(11):1027–1030.

26. Murphy E, Kapur N, Webb R, Cooper J. Risk assessment following self-harm: Comparison of mental health nurses and psychiatrists. *J Adv Nurs.* 2011;67(1):127–139.

27. National Center for Injury Prevention and Control, Centers for Disease Control and Prevention. Unintentional all injury causes nonfatal emergency department visits and rates per 100,000 2018, United States, all races, both sexes, all ages. https://webappa.cdc.gov/cgi-bin/broker.exe. Updated 2020. Accessed September 1, 2020.

28. Inder KJ, Holliday EG, Handley TE, et al. Depression and risk of unintentional injury in rural communities—A longitudinal analysis of the Australian Rural Mental Health Study. *Int J Environ Res Public Health.* 2017;14(9):1080. doi:10.3390/ijerph14091080.

29. Jenness JL, Witt CE, Quistberg DA, et al. Association of physical injury and mental health: Results from the National Comorbidity Survey—Adolescent Supplement. *J Psychiatr Res.* 2017;92:101–107.

30. Wan JJ, Morabito DJ, Khaw L, Knudson MM, Dicker RA. Mental illness as an independent risk factor for unintentional injury and injury recidivism. *J Trauma.* 2006;61(6):1299–1304.

31. Asbridge M, Azagba S, Langille DB, Rasic D. Elevated depressive symptoms and adolescent injury: Examining associations by injury frequency, injury type, and gender. *BMC Public Health.* 2014;14:190.

32. Korniloff K, Häkkinen A, Koponen HJ, et al. Relationships between depressive symptoms and self-reported unintentional injuries: The cross-sectional population-based FIN-D2D survey. *BMC Public Health.* 2012;12:516.

33. Hung CI, Liu CY, Yang CH. Unintentional injuries among psychiatric outpatients with major depressive disorder. *PLoS One.* 2016;11(12):e0168202.

34. Centers for Disease Control and Prevention, National Center for Injury Prevention and Control. 10 leading causes of death, United States 2018, all races, both sexes. https://webappa.cdc.gov/cgi-bin/broker.exe. Updated 2020. Accessed 09/01, 2020.

35. Rui P, Okeyode T. National Ambulatory Medical Care Survey: 2016 national summary tables (Table 17). 2016. Accessed February 25, 2021.

9
Broadening Our View of Risk

Now that we have discussed the need for improving approaches to risk identification and the importance of explicitly considering unintentional harm, we detail the rationale and evidence for the set of risks considered to be vital to comprehensive care.

As per the discussion regarding unintentional harm, each sphere of risk needs to be considered from both an intended and an unintended perspective. The only exception is suicide because its definition requires intended death as an outcome of the actions. Homicide also requires intent in most jurisdictions worldwide but can include death caused by recklessness and criminal negligence. Consequently, some homicides can be considered unintentional.

The set of risks that we address captures those most pressing that are associated with mental disorders and addiction. We discuss each area of risk separately and elaborate on the evidence for its inclusion. This finite set is also helpful when used as a list to check that specific risks are not overlooked throughout the duration people are in care.

Child Safety

Globally, most jurisdictions have legislation and agencies for child protection, although the definitions of child differ according to age. Critically, the younger the child, the more vulnerable they are and the greater the impact of inadequate care on their development. Despite legislation and the impact of compromised care, clinicians are often reluctant to address child well-being with their adult clients for fear of being intrusive or causing their clients additional distress. In addition to reluctance, clinicians may fail to recognize that a client's children are at risk of harm because the patient appears to have no intent to hurt them. Unintentional harm to children, however, is common.

Independent of intent at the time, harm toward others performed during the active phase of an illness is a profound source of suffering to our clients and persists beyond the illness. By failing to address the well-being of children under our patients' care, we are failing to address our patients' well-being.

A case that came before the courts in Canada serves to illustrate a parent's perspective on the issue of child protection. Despite its appearance in the public domain, details of the events were altered in the following description to preserve privacy.

A case attracted media attention when a woman being treated for a mood disorder brought a civil suit against both her family physician and her psychiatrist. At the time of the events, the woman was married and on leave from her career to raise the couple's 3-year-old daughter. The suit was successful.

The patient suffocated her daughter with a pillow. She then attempted to end her own life but was resuscitated by first responders. The husband came upon the bloody and messy scene in the morning when he checked in on his family before leaving for work. In the plaintiff's statement, she described the experience of persistently hearing her daughter's muffled cries 5 years after the event and of ongoing grief, guilt, and self-loathing.

Prior to the tragedy, both providers were aware that the patient was experiencing thoughts of ending her life but did not ask questions regarding potential homicide or other risks to the child. The clinicians argued that they had not referred the case to child protection services because they did not consider the child to be at risk and were concerned the patient's feelings of shame and worthlessness would worsen, further increasing her risk of suicide. They were wrong. Both the psychiatrist and the family physician were found at fault for failing to report the case to child protection services.

The best estimate is that an average of 500 children are killed by parents in the United States annually.[1] Unintentional death is even more frequent. In the fiscal year 2017, a national estimate in the United States reported that 1,720 children died from abuse and neglect.[2] This represents 33 children per week.

Clinicians tend to be anchored on acts of commission when thinking about risk, missing acts of omission and their significant impact. The relative contribution of acts of omission is reflected in the detailed data collected on childhood victims of maltreatment. In 2017, the Administration for Children and Families in the United States estimated 674,000 children were confirmed victims of maltreatment, 74.9% of these through neglect (acts of omission). That is more than half a million children in a single year harmed through neglect—almost 10,000 per week. Although these figures are not limited to cases involving active mental disorders, the American Society for the Positive Care of Children reported that one-third to two-thirds of maltreatment cases involve substance use.[3]

Numerous studies throughout the world consistently find that the number of children being cared for by parents with mental disorders is enormous and that these children are also at greater risk of suffering injury. In the United

Kingdom, 23.2% of mothers who have children younger than age 16 years struggle with mental illness.[4] A study of Canadian children younger than age 12 years cared for by parents with mental disorders found that for 17% of these children, the affected parent was the sole caregiver.[5] Viewed from a different perspective, a New Zealand study found that sole parents were two and a half times more likely to be suffering from a mental disorder compared with partnered parents.[6]

The obvious question is whether parental mental disorders are associated with increased risk of injury in their children. Even when solely dependent on maternal reports for information, maternal mental health problems were related to an increased risk of subsequent injury in children aged 3–11 years. This relationship was especially strong for children with multiple injuries.[7] A Swedish study of more than 1.5 million children compared those whose parents had a mental disorder to children whose parents did not. This study included both parents and found an increased risk in children aged 0–17 years, with children 0–1 year being at greatest risk.[8] The risk of injury from violence was approximately double that of unintentional injury, but the risk of unintentional transportation injuries increased as children aged. The severity of mental disorder symptoms is important. In studies of maternal depression, symptom severity correlated with an increasing risk of injury to children.[9,10]

It is likely that the available data on attempted killing and maltreatment by parents underestimate such events and that it is easy for clinicians to be unaware, as illustrated in the following case.

A woman in her early 50s, being treated by one of the authors for a recurring mood disorder with psychotic features, revealed unremitting guilt and nightmares. She only disclosed the content of the nightmares and intrusive memories after 7 years of familiarity with a treating clinician. She disclosed that she had attempted to drown her young children in the bathtub three times over 2 years. Although she was in active treatment at the time of the events, child protection services were never enlisted to assess the adequacy of her care when her children were at their most vulnerable ages.

The intention of the events was known only to the patient. Even the children were unaware of the mother's intention despite the violence of the acts. At the time of the attempted drownings, both children were younger than age 5 years, and neither child had any recollection of the events despite memories of other incidents at older ages.

At the time of the client's revelation, both children were in their 30s and still living in the parental home. The client also felt profound guilt that the attempted drownings and other forms of maltreatment, during her periods of illness, were responsible for both children struggling with severe mental illness. In the absence of the patient's revelations, there would have been no knowledge that these events had taken place. We doubt that this is a unique case.

Child protection laws, in most jurisdictions, mandate clinicians to report suspicion that a child is at risk. The evidence warrants such suspicions when clinicians have identified that a client is a parent of a child and especially when the child(ren) is younger, the client is a single parent, and symptoms are severe. The need to legislate reporting reminds us that we are reluctant to do so. It may be less uncomfortable for clinicians to conceptualize a report to child protection services as a referral for direct assessment of risk within the home environment. The previous cases also serve to remind clinicians that the involvement of child protection services is in the best interest of both the children and the client as parent.

Other Dependents

Many jurisdictions also have laws that require reporting of suspected abuse, neglect, or exploitation of vulnerable adults. Concern extends beyond legal requirements to cue the clinician's attention to the client's caregiving roles and identify related deficits. The issues discussed previously with respect to children are applicable to vulnerable adults, although data related to the mistreatment of vulnerable adults are difficult to find.

Conspicuously, information on the mistreatment of pets and other animals is easier to find. We include pets as dependents because of the large correlation between pet mistreatment and both domestic violence and child abuse. For instance, the Humane Society of the United States reports that 71% of domestic violence and 88% of child abuse cases include abuse of pets.[11] Therefore, inquiring about pets and exploring their care and treatment provide information with implications beyond the well-being of the pets. This includes alerting clinicians to an adult client's risk of being mistreated within a relationship with a person who abuses pets.

Motor Vehicles

This category includes the operation of vehicles for both personal and occupational purposes. The importance of identifying risk relating to motorized vehicles is reflected in the rates of injury and death resulting from motor vehicle accidents (MVAs).[12-15] Annually in the United States, approximately

3 million people are nonfatally injured in motor vehicle crashes. Beyond injury, more than 100 people per day die from motor vehicle injuries in the United States, totaling 36,560 people in 2018.[16]

Having a mental disorder alone (with or without a substance use disorder) has been repeatedly found to increase the odds of sustaining a motor vehicle-related injury.[12-15] However, alcohol and other substance use are massive contributors to MVAs and especially fatalities.[13,17-24] According to the U.S. National Highway Traffic Safety Administration, 10,511 deaths were formally attributed to alcohol intoxication in 2018 as verified by the operator having a blood alcohol concentration of 0.08 g/dL or greater.[25] Lower blood alcohol levels starting at 0.01 g/dL have also been shown to dramatically increase the severity of MVAs.[24] Consequently, alcohol use was implicated in one-third of all MVA deaths in the United States in 2018. These statistics do not include the impact of hangover, withdrawal, or other alcohol-related impairments on judgment, sustained attention, and reaction time. The impact of substances other than alcohol is also not reflected in these figures.

The extent to which providers overlook motor vehicle operation as a risk is unknown. In regions that mandate clinicians to inform the appropriate licensing bodies, rates of reporting unsafe drivers are much lower than predicted by the prevalence of mental disorders and addictions. Mandatory or permissible reporting provides clinicians with a mechanism of intervention that is more robust than simply informing patients about the risks. Prudence is difficult to impart, and the ubiquity of the confidence bias diminishes its influence. People believe they are excellent drivers, even when impaired, and that it is sufficient to "drive carefully."

Suicide

Unlike the other risks discussed in this chapter, suicide is addressed regularly in mental health research, has attracted health system attention, and most disciplines provide some teaching around it. According to the Centers for Disease Control and Prevention (CDC) WISQARS Leading Causes of Death Reports, in 2018, suicide was the 10th leading cause of death in the United States, claiming the lives of 48,344 people.[26] However, as discussed in previous chapters, clinician effectiveness in predicting suicide and reducing its contribution to death is poor.

Mitigating suicide is an enormous cognitive challenge for clinicians. Due to the prolonged period of risk over the course of active mental disorders, it is easy to become less vigilant and to allow mitigating interventions to wane.

Consequently, our approach is intended to cue the clinician to the risk of death by suicide throughout the entire course of management.

Homicide

It is beyond the scope of this book to provide details on the legal definition of homicide across different jurisdictions. As noted previously, however, most districts define homicide as involving some form of intent but may include recklessness and criminal negligence. We include homicide in the approach because it is easy for clinicians to overlook it and its profound consequences to both our patients and victims. In addition, our clients' family members and other loved ones are the most vulnerable and frequent victims. It is also a topic that clinicians are likely to feel uncomfortable asking about; that patients are likely to feel ashamed or guarded about; and that families, when interviewed about the risk of homicide, may be dismissive or angry about. Consequently, there are many disincentives for clinicians to explore the risk of homicide. We need a prompt to encourage its exploration or at least to remind us that we have not done it.

Suicide + Homicide

We have decided to cue clinicians to homicide paired with suicide in our approach because of the frequency of this combined tragedy and the tendency for clinicians to become anchored on singular issues. It is easy for the risk of suicide to pull the clinician's attention away from additional risks of harm, such as thoughts of killing others on route to suicide. Although families are at greatest risk, clinicians should also consider workplaces and neighbors. A sobering reminder of how easy it is to become anchored on one or the other of suicide and homicide is illustrated by the following case.

A resident, while being supervised by one of the authors, assessed an elderly retired gentleman in an emergency department. Mr. Y had been asked by his family doctor to be assessed for a possible relapse of depression with psychotic features. After presenting the case to the supervisor, the resident asked how to best respond to questions concerning the limits of confidentiality when asked by patients during an assessment. A brief discussion about the limits of confidentiality ensued, and then the supervisor asked what had prompted the patient's request for clarification. The trainee had not inquired into the patient's reason for asking. The supervisor returned with the resident to finalize the assessment and learned that Mr. Y was a retired security professional. They spent time explaining in detail the limits to confidentiality, including the extent of information that could be shared in each scenario and to whom. Following this explanation and answering the patient's additional questions, the supervisor reflected to Mr. Y that his question for clarification was common and sometimes asked by people who wish to discuss a sensitive topic. Mr. Y nodded his head slowly and went on to share realizations about his daughter-in-law that had been crystalizing over the previous weeks. He was certain that his grandchildren were in danger. He recognized that his beliefs about his daughter-in-law would probably not be believed by authorities because neither his wife nor his son believed him. Mr. Y concluded that the only solution was that he protect the grandchildren himself by removing their mother from the picture. The supervisor and resident established that Mr. Y had developed a plan to stab the daughter-in-law to death the next day.

The supervisor and resident became preoccupied with the details of the story and seeking consultation on whether duty to warn applied to the case or if it could be delayed during the period of involuntary hospital admission. When the team returned to speak with Mr. Y, he was informed of the decision to admit him to hospital involuntarily. He argued and informed the team that he would be contacting his lawyer and appealing every step of the process. Mr. Y then asked if he could be excused to use the restroom. As the resident was accompanying the patient, a large bottle of assorted sedatives and fentanyl slipped from within Mr. Y's track pants onto the floor. It was learned that Mr. Y was going to ingest the pills in the bathroom where he would not be seen, with the intent of ending his life. Both supervisor and resident realized that they had become so intrigued by the issue of the unexpected homicide plan that they neglected to consider the potential for suicide.

You may be thinking that it does not make sense that the patient would attempt to end his life prior to executing his plan to kill his daughter-in-law. We tend to use logic and linear thinking in our assessments, but mental disorders are neither linear nor logical.

Injury

Injury is much more common than death. Injury can be intentional, but the vast majority is unintentional, as revealed in the data provided previously. Because the risk of injury overlaps with the risk of unintentional death, this category thus includes injury with both fatal and nonfatal consequences.

Iatrogenic factors such as treatments that increase risk of various types of accidents can also result in injury and consequently require attention.[13,27,28]

Self-Care

Here, self-care primarily refers to basic nutrition, hygiene, self-safety, and attending to personal health needs. Deficient self-care can result in harm that is unlikely to be considered an injury or otherwise emphasized. For instance, the failure to follow-up on critical medical visits and poor management of chronic illness such as diabetes, respiratory diseases, heart disease, and so on are conditions that can accrue to death and contribute to years of life lost in persons with mental disorders.[29-34] Beyond death, lack of self-care can result in serious end organ damage and risk toward others, such as the impact of medical conditions on operating a motor vehicle, child care, and other responsibilities. Furthermore, we must consider the contribution of medical conditions to exacerbating the client's mental disorder or complicating its treatment.

Victimization and Harm Elicited

This risk of harm is especially easy to overlook and may be unfamiliar to many readers. This category also refers to situations in which a person's behavior elicits a response from others—including animals—in which they suffer non-fatal or fatal injury. We do not denote this risk exclusively as "victimization" because it does not capture the full scope of the risk. For instance, a person with a mental disorder may act with the *intent* of eliciting harm from others or may sustain harm while assaulting others. We illustrate, however, the disproportionate vulnerability to victimization when a person has symptoms of a mental disorder.

Harm can be elicited from others in multiple scenarios—for instance, transgressing rules and resisting redirection, aggravating others in the home or in public, when others must defend themselves from the client, during the process of an involuntary admission, while enforcing involuntary treatments, and so on. Many people with mental disorders are also more likely to be in close proximity to others with mental disorders, increasing the potential for reciprocal provocation.

Having a mental disorder or symptoms of one increases the probability of being victimized. This risk is not exclusively linked to psychoses or overt behaviors, although persons with psychotic disorders are almost five times more likely to be victims of violence.[35] The risk of sexual violence is particularly high in people who suffer serious mental illness, with a sixfold greater risk.[36] Studies also suggest that individuals with mental disorders have double the chance of being assaulted by various means: physical violence, with a weapon, robbery, sexual assault, partner and family violence and witnessing severe violence.[37,38] To be clear, people with alcohol use disorders are also at greater risk of violent and psychological victimization.[35,39]

We illustrate this risk of harm with two examples of common events, one of which is notorious.

Will, a 22-year-old athletic man, is brought to his local hospital by his parents due to several concerns. Will suddenly dropped out of college, where he had a baseball scholarship, and in the past several weeks has become completely withdrawn. In addition, in the past week, he has been walking throughout the house at night and his father has found him looking out windows and doors with his lucky bat on his shoulder. The parents report that during the past few days, Will has stopped eating and is expressing that his life is finished.

At the hospital, Will is minimally communicative. The only information that the team can elicit is that Will is frightened, convinced his life is over and that his situation is hopeless. The parents deny that their son's behavior is causing them concern for their safety. Will refuses to be admitted for continued assessment, but the decision is to proceed with an involuntary admission. During this process, Will becomes terrified and physically assaults several hospital staff who were attempting to prevent his departure. Will ultimately escapes barefoot and wearing nothing but a hospital gown.

Out of the hospital, Will runs to a convenience store, in which he grabs a pair of scissors and a small baseball bat all the while threatening others to stay away. The police are called, but their attempts to de-escalate the situation verbally and by using a Taser to subdue Will are unsuccessful. He charges the officers with both bat and scissors. The police defend themselves and their community by shooting the patient. Paramedics on the scene are unable to revive the young man and he succumbs to his injuries. This is an example of harm elicited from others and, as can be seen, was not intended by the patient nor the police services.

Let's shift to an ambulatory case.

You have been treating Millie for 6 months with a working diagnosis of Tourette's syndrome and obsessive–compulsive disorder. One of her vocal tics is to mutter "asshole." Usually this is not a problem because Millie has developed the ability to inhibit the tic until she can do it privately. On her way to see her clinician one morning, she is startled by a group of three people appearing from behind a concrete pillar in a subway station. To her horror, Millie mutters "asshole" several times before she can inhibit herself. Despite her attempts to apologize and explain, the trio immediately begin to beat her. Millie arrives at your appointment late and clearly injured. You send her to the hospital, where she is assessed to have facial fractures and a broken rib.

Notorious events in this category are fatalities during police apprehensions of persons with mental disorders, although nonfatal injuries are far more common.[40–43] In most communities, police services and their officers have become burdened with a problem for which health care systems are more appropriately accountable. The police are often used as mental health's de facto ambulance service without thorough consideration, planning, training and resources. This places police services, the afflicted, their families, and communities at risk.

Work

In contrast to assessing performance, viewing work through a risk lens is concerned with identifying and mitigating the potential for injury and death. The consideration of job-related risks begins with inquiring about the person's workplace, job, and responsibilities. This is important whether the person is currently working or already on sick leave, although interventions are prioritized for those actively working.

Numerous international studies consistently find that mental disorders increase the likelihood and frequency of workplace injuries.[28,44–48] Studies from the United Kingdom suggest that up to 10% of workplace injuries are due to mental disorders or their pharmacotherapy.[28] The identification of workplace injuries due to pharmacotherapy adds to the importance of incorporating iatrogenic risks into a comprehensive risk approach.

In the United States in 2018, there were 5,250 fatal workplace injuries, with the greatest number categorized as transportation incidents.[49] Nonfatal injury and illness are much more common. In private industry alone, 2.8 million nonfatal injuries and illnesses were reported in 2018. Conservatively applying Palmer et al.'s[28] findings to U.S. data suggests 280,000 private industry injuries were due to mental disorders or their treatment in 2018.

The gravity of injuries in U.S. private industry is reflected in the 79,470 fractures and 5,920 amputations in 2018. With respect to risk in the workplace, we must also consider the nature of our clients' jobs and the potential for harm—for instance, the potential for harm from errors made by health care workers, military personnel, health inspectors, and mechanics. Similarly, we must consider clients with professional licenses, such as physicians, psychologists, lawyers, and accountants, and the potential for unintentional harm from errors.

Financial

Internationally, government offices, such as public trustees and guardians, which manage the financial affairs of people during periods of financial incapacity, agree that mental disorders wreak havoc on personal finances. This is especially true when individuals lack insight into their conditions. The mechanisms by which mental disorders impair financial management are varied and include impaired judgment, increased susceptibility to exploitation, losing or lending money to other people, making impulsive or unnecessary purchases, and spending limited funds on harmful drugs and alcohol. Insufficient funds can also start a cascade of harm on the person's health, social functioning, and risk of homelessness.[50] The problem is worse when the afflicted person has no discretionary income because the margin for error disappears.

Financial risk also includes harm to others. For instance, people with bipolar disorder, addictions, and gambling disorders can lay waste to family savings and assets. In the United States, there is the additional factor that more than a half million people per year declare bankruptcy due to medical costs and sick time off work. The prolonged periods of disability associated with mental disorders accrue to enormous reductions in income. Even in countries with publicly funded health care, such as Canada, loss of job, periods of inability to work, and cost of medication have serious consequences for the financial status of persons with mental disorders and their families.

The enormous complexity of factors contributing to financial harm exceeds the scope of clinical practice. Identification and thorough assessment of the risk of overspending or poor financial decisions during the active phase of illness should be the minimum. Interventions such as temporary periods of formal incapacity with transfer of financial management to trustees or family can be critical in preventing financial devastation or mitigating losses. These should be consistently used when indicated.

Housing

Housing is important to use as a cue because of the robust literature that links it to health and because people with mental disorders and addiction are at high risk of losing housing due to inadequate income, impaired activities of daily living, behavior toward others, periods of incarceration in hospital or prison, and certain psychotic symptoms. Another factor is that the age of onset of most disorders covers developmental periods when people first begin living independently, and thus some people with mental disorders may have never established a foothold in permanent housing.

A critical reason for paying attention to housing is to reduce the probability of experiencing homelessness. Homelessness is associated with increased rates of harm, including facial fractures as a consequence of being assaulted,[51] death from all causes, and a 7.6-fold greater risk of homicide.[52] Within the population of people with mental and substance use disorders, those who are homeless have a 3-fold greater risk of death than those that are not. This risk is highest for females, who have a mortality rate ratio as high as 107.[53,54] Homelessness also increases the risk of intentional self-harm,[55,56] victimization,[57,58] legal incarceration,[58,59] and rates of hospitalization.[60]

In addition to homelessness is the issue of clients being housed in units that match their level of needed support. This overlaps with self-care, and related interventions are likely to be determined by the mutability of impairments. For instance, if the inability to care for self is due to a phase of illness that will respond to treatment, then it may be that the solution is hospitalization followed by outreach services. However, if the impairment persists beyond a phase of illness and is prolonged or permanent, then the intervention may necessitate supportive housing.

Firearms

Our discussion of firearms is guided by the same apolitical client-centered framework we use in considering harm related to work, motor vehicles, and other factors. Research suggests that in 2017, 30% of American citizens (97.5 million) owned a gun and 42% (136.5 million) lived in a household with a gun.[61] Consequently, clinicians must consider firearm-related risk with all their patients.

Figures 9.1 and 9.2 illustrate the involvement of firearms in various types of death in the United States and Canada, respectively. We chose to use pie charts to avoid the confound of dramatically different population sizes but also to reveal similarities in types of firearm deaths despite the differences in gun laws. Evidence strongly suggests an overrepresentation of people with mental disorders on both ends of the gun.[62-65] The greatest risk, however, is suicide by firearm, which greatly exceeds homicide in both Canada and the

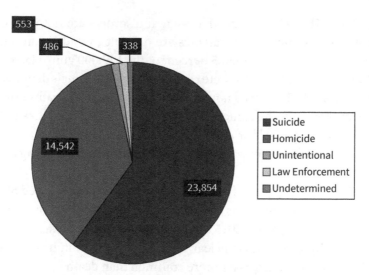

Figure 9.1 Firearm deaths in the United States in 2017 for all ages, sex, and races.
Source: Data from Centers for Disease Control and Prevention's WONDER online database.

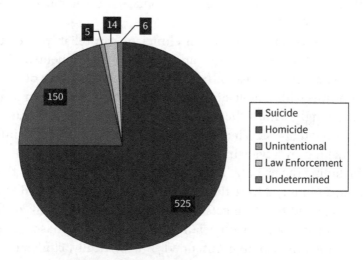

Figure 9.2 Firearm deaths in Canada in 2018 for all ages, sex, and races.
Source: Data from Statistics Canada (2020) Table 13-10-0392-01 Deaths and age-specific mortality rates, by selected group causes (formerly CANSIM Table 102-0551). https://www150.statcan.gc.ca/t1/tbl1/en/tv.action?pid=1310039201. Data for law enforcement–related deaths are from List of killings by law enforcement officers in Canada Wikipedia (https://en.wikipedia.org/wiki/List_of_killings_by_law_enforcement_officers_in_Canada; accessed July 5, 2020).

United States. This is not to say that mental disorders are not implicated in firearm-related homicide, but statistics are difficult to find. In an online article, one estimate is "fewer than 5 percent of the 120,000 gun-related killings in the U.S. between 2001–2010 were carried out by individuals diagnosed with a mental illness."[66] This would nonetheless represent 6,000 deaths during that period. Consequently, the clinician needs to be attentive to the risk of firearm injury whether it is to self or others, intentional or unintentional. Providers also need to consider the impact of treatments on the safe handling and operation of a firearm.

In 2017, the total number of firearm-related deaths in the United States was 39,773, but of equal interest is the mitigation of the impact of nonfatal injury. The CDC's estimate for 2015 totaled 84,997 nonfatal firearm injuries and 36,252 deaths by guns.[67] It is unclear what proportion of injuries were unintended, but nonfatal injury is far more common than death.

It is extremely difficult to obtain nonfatal firearm-related injuries in Canada because Statistics Canada does not collect this information. We did, however, find peer-reviewed studies for Ontario, the province in which 39% of Canada's population reside. These data are for a period of 17 years from April 2002 to April 2019 and revealed there were 7,746 nonfatal firearm injuries in persons aged 16 years or older.[68]

There is no mechanism by which clinicians can reliably interrupt access to guns in the United States and Canada. Consequently, clinicians will need to address the risk of firearm-related harm using other strategies. This begins with establishing the client's accessibility to firearms and acting accordingly within the laws of each jurisdiction to reduce access during the period of risk. The clinician can optimize the client's informed decision making by reviewing with them the risk of harm to self and others, including the fact that damage done by firearms is easier to inflict, more rapid, and more severe than damage from other potential weapons, such as knives and blunt objects. Because most people think of firearm injuries as intentional, it is especially important to emphasize that injuries and deaths can also be unintended. Pragmatically, clinicians should collaborate with clients in developing personalized strategies to mitigate firearm-related harm.

With respect to risks to family members such as children, an important and pragmatic mitigating strategy can focus on safe storage of the firearm. Alcohol misuse by parents in households with firearms has been studied by several groups, and findings reveal an increased risk of unsafe storage in households in which the parent misuses alcohol.[69,70]

If nothing else, learning that clients have access to firearms should increase the clinician's urgency in treating the mental disorder and substance misuse. This translates into more frequent follow-up, increased vigilance for symptom change, more rapid modification of interventions when treatment response is unimpressive, connection to community resources, and enlisting the assistance of child protection services as needed. Identification and management of alcohol misuse are particularly urgent due to alcohol's amplification of both intentional and unintentional firearm injuries.[71]

Summary

In this chapter, we identified critical areas of harm relevant to mental disorders. We discussed the rationale and evidence supporting their inclusion as a part of a thorough approach to risk identification. In Chapter 10, we describe aspects of impaired functioning and critical symptoms that relate to risk of harm and also describe the structure of a novel approach to risk identification.

References

1. Criss D. A parent killing a child happens more often than we think. https://www.cnn.com/2017/07/07/health/filicide-parents-killing-kids-stats-trnd/index.html. Updated 2017. Accessed August 31, 2020.
2. Administration for Children and Families. 28th edition of the Child Maltreatment Report. https://www.acf.hhs.gov/media/press/2019/child-abuse-neglect-data-released. Published 2019. Accessed August 31, 2020.
3. American Society for the Positive Care of Children. Child abuse statistics. https://americanspcc.org/child-abuse-statistics. Accessed August 31, 2020.
4. Abel KM, Hope H, Swift E, et al. Prevalence of maternal mental illness among children and adolescents in the UK between 2005 and 2017: A national retrospective cohort analysis. *Lancet Public Health*. 2019;4(6):e291–e300.
5. Bassani DG, Padoin CV, Philipp D, Veldhuizen S. Estimating the number of children exposed to parental psychiatric disorders through a national health survey. *Child Adolesc Psychiatry Ment Health*. 2009;3(1):6.
6. Tobias M, Gerritsen S, Kokaua J, Templeton R. Psychiatric illness among a nationally representative sample of sole and partnered parents in New Zealand. *Aust N Z J Psychiatry*. 2009;43(2):136–144.
7. Hope S, Deighton J, Micali N, Law C. Maternal mental health and childhood injury: Evidence from the UK Millennium Cohort Study. *Arch Dis Child*. 2019;104(3):268–274.
8. Nevriana A, Pierce M, Dalman C, et al. Association between maternal and paternal mental illness and risk of injuries in children and adolescents: Nationwide register based cohort study in Sweden. *BMJ*. 2020;369:m853.

9. Schwebel DC, Brezausek CM. Chronic maternal depression and children's injury risk. *J Pediatr Psychol.* 2008;33(10):1108–1116.

10. Phelan K, Khoury J, Atherton H, Kahn RS. Maternal depression, child behavior, and injury. *Inj Prev.* 2007;13(6):403–408. http://injuryprevention.bmj.com/content/13/6/403.abstract. doi:10.1136/ip.2006.014571.

11. The Humane Society of the United States. Animal cruelty facts and stats: What to know about abuse victims and legislative trends. https://www.humanesociety.org/resources/animal-cruelty-facts-and-stats. Updated 2020. Accessed October 4, 2020.

12. Asbridge M, Azagba S, Langille DB, Rasic D. Elevated depressive symptoms and adolescent injury: Examining associations by injury frequency, injury type, and gender. *BMC Public Health.* 2014;14:190.

13. Modén B, Ohlsson H, Merlo J, Rosvall M. Psychotropic drugs and accidents in Scania, Sweden. *Eur J Public Health.* 2012;22(5):726–732.

14. Shadloo B, Motevalian A, Rahimi-Movaghar V, et al. Psychiatric disorders are associated with an increased risk of injuries: Data from the Iranian Mental Health Survey (IranMHS). *Iran J Public Health.* 2016;45(5):623–635.

15. Wan JJ, Morabito DJ, Khaw L, Knudson MM, Dicker RA. Mental illness as an independent risk factor for unintentional injury and injury recidivism. *J Trauma.* 2006;61(6):1299–1304.

16. Insurance Institute for Highway Safety in the USA. Fatality facts 2018, yearly snapshot. https://www.iihs.org/topics/fatality-statistics/detail/yearly-snapshot. Updated 2019. Accessed August 31, 2020.

17. Schlotthauer AE, Guse CE, Brixey S, Corden TE, Hargarten SW, Layde PM. Motor vehicle crashes associated with alcohol: Child passenger injury and restraint use. *Am J Prev Med.* 2011;40(3):320–323.

18. Sauber-Schatz EK, Ederer DJ, Dellinger AM, Baldwin GT. Vital signs: Motor vehicle injury prevention—United States and 19 comparison countries. *MMWR Morb Mortal Wkly Rep.* 2016;65(26):672–677.

19. Redelmeier DA, Manzoor F. Life-threatening alcohol-related traffic crashes in adverse weather: A double-matched case–control analysis from Canada. *BMJ Open.* 2019;9(3):e024415.

20. Papalimperi AH, Athanaselis SA, Mina AD, Papoutsis II, Spiliopoulou CA, Papadodima SA. Incidence of fatalities of road traffic accidents associated with alcohol consumption and the use of psychoactive drugs: A 7-year survey (2011–2017). *Exp Ther Med.* 2019;18(3):2299–2306.

21. Khanjani N, Mousavi M, Dehghanian A, Jahani Y, Soori H. The role of drug and alcohol use and the risk of motor vehicle crashes in Shiraz, Iran, 2014: A case–crossover study. *Traffic Inj Prev.* 2017;18(6):573–576.

22. Huang Y, Liu C, Pressley JC. Child restraint use and driver screening in fatal crashes involving drugs and alcohol. *Pediatrics.* 2016;138(3):e20160319. doi:10.1542/peds.2016-0319.

23. Hall AJ, Bixler D, Helmkamp JC, Kraner JC, Kaplan JA. Fatal all-terrain vehicle crashes: Injury types and alcohol use. *Am J Prev Med.* 2009;36(4):311–316.

24. Phillips DP, Brewer KM. The relationship between serious injury and blood alcohol concentration (BAC) in fatal motor vehicle accidents: BAC = 0.01% is associated with significantly more dangerous accidents than BAC = 0.00%. *Addiction.* 2011;106(9):1614–1622.

25. National Center for Statistics and Analysis. 2018 fatal motor vehicle crashes: Overview. Traffic Safety Facts Research Note, Report No. DOT HS 812 826. https://crashstats.nhtsa.dot.gov/Api/Public/ViewPublication/812826. Accessed July 12, 2020.

26. Centers for Disease Control and Prevention, National Center for Injury Prevention and Control. 10 leading causes of death, United States 2018, all races, both sexes. https://webappa.cdc.gov/cgi-bin/broker.exe. Updated 2020. Accessed September 1, 2020.

27. Wadsworth EJ, Moss SC, Simpson SA, Smith AP. Psychotropic medication use and accidents, injuries and cognitive failures. *Hum Psychopharmacol.* 2005;20(6):391–400.

28. Palmer KT, D'Angelo S, Harris EC, Linaker C, Coggon D. The role of mental health problems and common psychotropic drug treatments in accidental injury at work: A case–control study. *Occup Environ Med.* 2014;71(5):308–312.

29. Wu CY, Chang CK, Hayes RD, Broadbent M, Hotopf M, Stewart R. Clinical risk assessment rating and all-cause mortality in secondary mental healthcare: The South London and Maudsley NHS Foundation Trust Biomedical Research Centre (SLAM BRC) case register. *Psychol Med.* 2012;42(8):1581–1590.

30. Pearson S, Nash T, Ireland V. Depression symptoms in people with diabetes attending outpatient podiatry clinics for the treatment of foot ulcers. *J Foot Ankle Res.* 2014;7(1):47.

31. Turner A, Hochschild A, Burnett J, Zulfiqar A, Dyer CB. High prevalence of medication non-adherence in a sample of community-dwelling older adults with adult protective services-validated self-neglect. *Drugs Aging.* 2012;29(9):741–749.

32. Dong X, Simon M. Prevalence of elder self-neglect in a Chicago Chinese population: The role of cognitive physical and mental health. *Geriatr Gerontol Int.* 2016;16(9):1051–1062.

33. Gonzalez JS, Safren SA, Delahanty LM, et al. Symptoms of depression prospectively predict poorer self-care in patients with type 2 diabetes. *Diabet Med.* 2008;25(9):1102–1107.

34. Lunghi C, Zongo A, Moisan J, Grégoire JP, Guénette L. Factors associated with antidiabetic medication non-adherence in patients with incident comorbid depression. *J Diabetes Complications.* 2017;31(7):1200–1206.

35. Morgan VA, Morgan F, Galletly C, Valuri G, Shah S, Jablensky A. Sociodemographic, clinical and childhood correlates of adult violent victimisation in a large, national survey sample of people with psychotic disorders. *Soc Psychiatry Psychiatr Epidemiol.* 2016;51(2):269–279.

36. Khalifeh H, Oram S, Osborn D, Howard LM, Johnson S. Recent physical and sexual violence against adults with severe mental illness: A systematic review and meta-analysis. *Int Rev Psychiatry.* 2016;28(5):433–451.

37. Bhavsar V, Dean K, Hatch SL, MacCabe JH, Hotopf M. Psychiatric symptoms and risk of victimisation: A population-based study from southeast London. *Epidemiol Psychiatr Sci.* 2019;28(2):168–178.

38. Khalifeh H, Moran P, Borschmann R, et al. Domestic and sexual violence against patients with severe mental illness. *Psychol Med.* 2015;45(4):875–886.

39. Christ C, Ten Have M, de Graaf R, et al. Mental disorders and the risk of adult violent and psychological victimisation: A prospective, population-based study. *Epidemiol Psychiatr Sci.* 2019;29:e13.

40. Kesic D, Thomas SD, Ogloff JR. Mental illness among police fatalities in Victoria 1982–2007: Case linkage study. *Aust N Z J Psychiatry.* 2010;44(5):463–468.

41. Kesic D, Thomas SD, Ogloff JR. Estimated rates of mental disorders in, and situational characteristics of, incidents of nonfatal use of force by police. *Soc Psychiatry Psychiatr Epidemiol.* 2013;48(2):225–232.

42. Holloway-Beth A, Forst L, Lippert J, Brandt-Rauf S, Freels S, Friedman L. Risk factors associated with legal interventions. *Inj Epidemiol.* 2016;3(1).

43. Farkas K, Matthay EC, Rudolph KE, Goin DE, Ahern J. Mental and substance use disorders among legal intervention injury cases in California, 2005–2014. *Prev Med.* 2019;121:136–140.

44. Lefkowitz RY, Null DB, Slade MD, Redlich CA. Injury, illness, and mental health risks in United States domestic mariners. *J Occup Environ Med.* 2020;62(10):839–841.

45. Gerasimaviciute V, Bültmann U, Diamond PM, et al. Reciprocal associations between depression, anxiety and work-related injury. *Inj Prev.* 2019;26(6).

46. Gaspar FW, Jolivet DN, Wizner K, Schott F, Dewa CS. Pre-existing and new-onset depression and anxiety among workers with injury or illness work leaves. *J Occup Environ Med.* 2020;62(10):e567–e572.

47. Cherry N, Burstyn I, Beach J. Mental ill-health and second claims for work-related injury. *Occup Med (Lond).* 2012;62(6):462–465.

48. Kim J, Choi Y. Gender differences in the longitudinal association between work-related injury and depression. *Int J Environ Res Public Health.* 2016;13(11):1077. doi:10.3390/ijerph13111077.

49. Bureau of Labor Statistics. National census of fatal occupational injuries in 2018. USDL-19-2194:1–9. https://www.bls.gov/news.release/archives/cfoi_12172019.pdf. Published 2019. Accessed July 17, 2020.

50. Moore BA, Black AC, Rosen MI. Factors associated with money mismanagement among adults with severe mental illness and substance abuse. *Int J Ment Health Addict.* 2016;14(4):400–409.

51. Nguyen AB, Grimes B, Neuhaus J, Pomerantz JH. A cross-sectional study of the association between homelessness and facial fractures. *Plast Reconstr Surg Glob Open.* 2019;7(6):e2254.

52. Schinka JA, Leventhal KC, Lapcevic WA, Casey R. Mortality and cause of death in younger homeless veterans. *Public Health Rep.* 2018;133(2):177–181.

53. Feodor Nilsson S, Laursen TM, Hjorthøj C, Nordentoft M. Homelessness as a predictor of mortality: An 11-year register-based cohort study. *Soc Psychiatry Psychiatr Epidemiol.* 2018;53(1):63–75.

54. Feodor Nilsson S, Hjorthøj CR, Erlangsen A, Nordentoft M. Suicide and unintentional injury mortality among homeless people: A Danish nationwide register-based cohort study. *Eur J Public Health.* 2014;24(1):50–56.

55. Pluck G, Lee KH, Parks RW. Self-harm and homeless adults. *Crisis.* 2013;34(5):363–366.

56. Barrett P, Griffin E, Corcoran P, O'Mahony MT, Arensman E. Self-harm among the homeless population in Ireland: A national registry-based study of incidence and associated factors. *J Affect Disord.* 2018;229:523–531.

57. Tong MS, Kaplan LM, Guzman D, Ponath C, Kushel MB. Persistent homelessness and violent victimization among older adults in the HOPE HOME study. *J Interpers Violence.* 2019:886260519850532.

58. Roy L, Crocker AG, Nicholls TL, Latimer EA, Ayllon AR. Criminal behavior and victimization among homeless individuals with severe mental illness: A systematic review. *Psychiatr Serv.* 2014;65(6):739–750.

59. Kouyoumdjian FG, Wang R, Mejia-Lancheros C, et al. Interactions between police and persons who experience homelessness and mental illness in Toronto, Canada: Findings from a prospective study. *Can J Psychiatry.* 2019;64(10):718–725.

60. Cheung A, Somers JM, Moniruzzaman A, et al. Emergency department use and hospitalizations among homeless adults with substance dependence and mental disorders. *Addict Sci Clin Pract.* 2015;10:17.

61. Pew Research Center. *America's Complex Relationship with Guns.* Pew Research Center; 2017.

62. Swanson JW, McGinty EE, Fazel S, Mays VM. Mental illness and reduction of gun violence and suicide: Bringing epidemiologic research to policy. *Ann Epidemiol.* 2015;25(5):366–376.

63. Swanson JW, Sampson NA, Petukhova MV, et al. Guns, impulsive angry behavior, and mental disorders: Results from the National Comorbidity Survey Replication (NCS-R). *Behav Sci Law.* 2015;33(2–3):199–212.

64. Rozel JS, Mulvey EP. The link between mental illness and firearm violence: Implications for social policy and clinical practice. *Annu Rev Clin Psychol.* 2017;13:445–469.

65. Pinals DA, Anacker L. Mental illness and firearms: Legal context and clinical approaches. *Psychiatr Clin North Am*. 2016;39(4):611–621.
66. Naprawa AZ. Mental illness and gun violence. *Berkley Wellness*. 2016. https://www. berkeleywellness.com/healthy-community/health-care-policy/article/mental-illness-really-behind-most-gun-violence. Accessed September 14, 2020.
67. Centers for Disease Control and Prevention, National Center for Health Statistics. Deaths: Final data for 2017. *Natl Vital Stat Rep*. 2019;68(9). https://www.cdc.gov/nchs/data/nvsr/nvsr68/nvsr68_09_tables-508.pdf. Accessed July 5, 2020.
68. Raza S, Thiruchelvam D, Redelmeier DA. Death and long-term disability after gun injury: A cohort analysis. *CMAJ Open*. 2020;8(3):E469–E478.
69. Morgan ER, Gomez A, Rivara FP, Rowhani-Rahbar A. Firearm storage and adult alcohol misuse among Washington state households with children. *JAMA Pediatr*. 2019;173(1):37–43.
70. Martin-Storey A, Prickett KC, Crosnoe R. Alcohol use and change over time in firearm safety among families with young children. *Drug Alcohol Depend*. 2018;186:187–192.
71. Branas CC, Han S, Wiebe DJ. Alcohol use and firearm violence. *Epidemiol Rev*. 2016;38(1):32–45.

10

A Novel Approach to Risk Identification

The Risk, Function, and Symptoms Approach

Ultimately, the goal of all diagnostic systems is to facilitate the reduction of mortality, morbidity, and suffering.[1,2] This too is the goal of developing an approach to comprehensive risk identification. The approach we propose simply bypasses the intermediate step of diagnosis and avoids the impact of diagnostic error on recognizing and addressing suffering related to harm and impairment. This approach integrates risk of harm (R), functional impairments (F), and critical symptoms (S). The symptom component of the RFS approach aligns with dimensional or phenomenological approaches.

The ideal approach to risk identification should reduce the clinician's susceptibility to prematurely narrow attention to specific risks with the consequence of missing others. It should begin with broad categories related to the client and others, followed by attention to functional impairments and then symptoms that may cue the physician to risks not otherwise identified. Assessment tools focused on specific risks in mental health, such as suicide and violence, are already available. However, they do not provide a cognitive framework for identifying a comprehensive set of high-impact risks, such as those we described in Chapter 9.

The proposed approach is organized into grids to facilitate data gathering and the organization of one's thoughts during and after the clinical interview to determine if any risks were missed. The framework deconstructs the array of gathered information into components to inform judgment and decision making. Furthermore, in keeping with the complex and fluctuating nature of mental disorders, the approach is intended to guide the clinician to consider risk throughout the duration of care rather than from a singular assessment.

A finite number of risks, functional impairments, and symptoms were delineated from morbidity and mortality data, the literature, broadly identified adverse events, concepts from judgment and decision making, clinical practice, program development, supervision of residents, and mentorship of health care providers. The categories of risk, impaired functioning, and symptoms can be considered independently or jointly. Knowing that the contents of the framework are finite may help reduce anxiety and the feeling of being overwhelmed that can accompany our work with clients. The schema is designed to limit cognitive load, organize thinking, reduce cognitive errors, and amplify information relevant to harm reduction. The approach is also designed to reduce overprecision in judgment. The hope is to decrease the probability of ignoring or missing key issues that must be addressed urgently or consistently.

The RFS approach is agnostic with respect to theories of mind and mental disorders. It endeavors to deal with "just the facts." It does not utilize interpretations, causal formulations, or other historical attempts to replace complexity and irreducible uncertainty with *understanding* or insight. However, in mental health care, clinicians are often dependent on inferences arising from the complex array of information. It is inevitable that the synthesis of data, and its gaps, will result in questions and suspicions. Consequently, in addition to categories of information that is "observed" or "reported," the approach includes a category denoted as "suspected." This encourages clinicians to make use of inferences but to explicitly recognize them as suspicions rather than facts.

The approach has undergone proof of concept through continuing education of health care providers and the training of family physician and psychiatry residents. It was adapted by a leading Canadian knowledge translation organization to create a tool for primary care providers.[3] The point-of-care tool, Keeping Your Patients Safe: A Guide to Primary Care Management of Mental Health and Addictions-Related Risks and Functional Impairment, has been downloaded 8,847 times as of February 22, 2021 (see Appendix 3). The approach has also been published in a peer-reviewed journal and used in clinical practice. Although it has not yet been empirically tested, it is a coherent approach, the feasibility and effectiveness of which can be investigated. Our experience with using the approach during the past decade is that it is easily applicable to all aspects of patient care and has improved users' effectiveness in reducing harm to patients. It is our hope that this book will stimulate further research into this approach to risk identification.

Risk of Harm

Harm is a term that is used in myriad ways in mental health care. When we refer to risk of *harm* as applied to the approach, we are limiting our focus to material harm that has a permanent or long-lasting impact through death or adds to impairment and/or suffering of the patient or others. Mitigating the probability of such harm and additional suffering is the priority.

An important question for any assessment tool relates to the issue of time pressures and the resistance clinicians have to structured tools of assessment. The emphasis on brevity tends to be prioritized in the development of such clinical tools. In our search for other broad approaches to risk, we found an interesting description of one designed to improve communication of identified risks across providers. The authors stated that "clinicians felt reassured by the fact that completion of RIF [Risk Identification Form] took less than a minute" (p. 370).[4] Reassurance and expediency do not necessarily translate into better outcomes. The prioritization of speed and ease in risk assessments is a concrete and poignant reflection of the discordance between the lip service paid to prioritizing risk assessment, in mental health, and the actual time and effort that we devote to it. The prolonged duration of mental disorders, even when being treated, provides clinicians with more than 1 minute to focus on reducing the probability our clients and others will suffer harm. Our clients and others sustain injury, disability, and death when we fail to adequately identify and respond to material risks, all of which generally last longer "than a minute."

We were otherwise unable to find published literature on existing approaches to comprehensive risk assessment in mental health care. However, we did find one focused on suicide using similar principles and decision-making concepts that guide our approach.[5] We thus concluded that no other such approach to multiple risks of harm currently exists.

The priority in developing our approach was not brevity but instead that it be thorough, aligned with evidence relating to clinician judgment, and respectful of the irreducible uncertainty and inevitable error inherent to risk management. This is not to dismiss the importance of ease of use and the time required to implement a clinical aid. However, if a tool does not improve a clinician's success in achieving their desired outcomes, ease of use is irrelevant, and the time spent is truly wasted.

A key aim is to decrease the cognitive demand on clinicians by reducing the number of variables to be considered during assessment and by organizing the information into intuitive chunks to optimize efficiency without compromising thoroughness. The transdiagnostic nature of the approach is intended to minimize the drain on cognitive resources by precluding the need for diagnostic certainty. Recognition of uncertainty, complexity, and their contribution to inevitable error is woven into the fabric of the approach. This is achieved by incorporating the interactions between risk of harm and impairment and explicating the contribution of unintended harm. In addition, clinicians are not required to make predictions about the probability of events by stratifying risks into low, medium, and high.

The flexibility of an approach is critical if it is to be applicable across settings and disciplines. The RFS approach was designed as such and can be used in a variety of ways, as a whole or in part. Once familiar with its use, the time it takes to utilize it is not onerous. We encourage the reader to try the approach, knowing that any modification or change to practice requires effort to adopt and time to assess its return on investment.

In brief, the structure of the approach is intended to aid clinician judgment and decision making by facilitating the comprehensive identification of potential harm (judgment), thus improving the accuracy and clarity of the information, and its gaps, employed in decision making. Clinicians will find that the approach clarifies candidate answers to the following questions:

1. What do I need to do now?
2. What do I need to do soon?
3. What do I need to pay attention to over time?

These three questions can help clinicians organize their thinking and decision making in terms of acuity and chronicity independent of diagnostic clarity. It helps them determine what aspects of the client's condition require immediate attention and what issues allow for the luxury of unhurried contemplation.

The Approach in Matrix Form

The approach is organized into three matrices consisting of one matrix each for risk of harm, impairment in functioning, and critical symptoms. Why not simply use checklists? Matrices make it easier to clarify relationships between variables. In addressing risks, the matrix helps highlight the kinds of risks and organizes them into categories that provide the clinician with a cognitive framework that has practical use for management. The matrix also facilitates the consideration of risks that are often forgotten or not considered. For impairment and symptoms, the matrices are organized according to how the information was received and assists the clinician in gauging its reliability and accuracy. This is intended to assist clinicians to modulate their degree of confidence in their judgments and is reminiscent of guidelines that categorize the level of evidence for their recommendations. We think the use of these matrices is elegant and improves the signal-to-noise ratio around the issues most salient to the person who is at risk. A description and explanation of the elements of each matrix, beginning with the risk matrix, follow.

The Risk Matrix

The RFS approach is comprehensive and consists of those risks with which we are familiar (suicide and violence) as well as those that go beyond the traditional literature and training. The set of risks that require vigilance were discussed in Chapter 9. The full set is listed here, with the risks that are not highlighted in training, clinical practice, and risk assessment tools shown in bold:

1. Child safety
2. **Other dependents**
3. **Motor vehicles**
4. Suicide
5. Homicide
6. **Suicide + homicide**
7. **Injury**
8. Self-care
9. **Victimization and harm elicited**
10. **Work**
11. **Financial**
12. **Housing**
13. **Firearms**
14. **Iatrogenic risks as a domain of risk**

In the matrix, each risk of harm is considered according to the person experiencing it (i.e., self or others) and the intentionality of the risk (i.e., intended, unintended, or iatrogenic). Regardless of intentionality, risk of harm can result from acts of omission or commission. Iatrogenic risk was judged to be an important risk to include in the matrix based on feedback from clinicians and malpractice data. Furthermore, it aligns with the ethical precept of nonmaleficence, central to all forms of health care, recognizing that many clinical decisions are associated with the potential for adverse events independent of error.

We have not emphasized acts of commission or omission as explicit subcategories in each cell of the matrix, in order to balance utility with cognitive burden. Nonetheless, it is important to keep acts of omission in mind—for instance, a person who stops eating or drinking due to profound anergia and amotivation. Such a case is an example of unintentional risk of harm to self through acts of omission in the form of not eating or drinking adequately. Even more likely to be missed are risks resulting in unintentional harm to others stemming from acts of omission.

Incorporating Intentional Versus Unintentional Harm

The approach's consideration of harm according to intentionality warrants further discussion. Using the example of death of a person with an active mental disorder illustrates the utility of this aspect of risk identification. For a death to be judged suicide requires that the deceased intended this outcome. Determining intent in the absence of available reports from the deceased is a difficult task. Furthermore, the impairments and symptoms associated with mental disorders can give rise to numerous mechanisms of death that are unintended, including acute deaths (e.g., workplace accident) or less acute deaths (e.g., failing to use insulin). Consequently, if we become anchored in exclusively considering risk of intentional death and fail to assess risk of death that is unintentional, our identification of potential harms will be incomplete. As we illustrated in Chapter 8, the frequency of unintentional harm such as death and injury far exceeds that of intentional harm.

The risk of unintended harm is not unique to mental health and occurs in association with many other types of illness in medicine. A patient with an unstable cardiac condition is at risk of causing death to themself or others unintentionally—for instance, suffering a cardiac event while driving. For this reason, many jurisdictions require that clinicians inform the patient and/or licensing body that the patient is not safe to operate a motor vehicle. I, We can also consider a parent with a treatment refractory seizure disorder alone at home with a toddler: While carrying the toddler down a set of stairs, the parent suffers a seizure. Risks in these other areas of health care, however, are reliably predicted by pathophysiology (e.g., cardiac death), and tend to be linear, and the sequelae are relatively easy to identify. The conditions usually come in a tidy package with the diagnoses being considered. Just unpack the box and there it is—etiology, pathophysiology, signs and symptoms, risks, diagnostic maneuvers, and treatment options. Risks that are not embedded within pathophysiology are less likely to enter the clinician's mind because they seem tangential to the disease—for example, the motor vehicle accident secondary to a cardiac event. However, such an event that results from reduced consciousness is linearly related to pathophysiology and should be expected. In mental health, most risks that are associated with mental disorders are nonlinear and frequently emerge from a context. The risks that must be considered in mental health do not come in a neat, orderly package, labeled with the diagnosis and pathophysiology.

With respect to unintentional harm toward others and considering acts of omission versus acts of commission, where would the clinician's greatest vulnerability be? Until proven otherwise, evidence related to human cognition, and clinician errors, predicts that we are most likely to miss the probability of harm to others that is unintentional and resulting from an act of omission—for instance, a toddler who wanders onto a road due to neglect by the caregiver while intoxicated.

In its current form, the risk matrix is composed of risks to self and/or others that may be intended, unintended, or iatrogenically induced, and it consists of the following areas: child safety—neglect/abuse, whether the patient is safe to operate a motor vehicle, suicide and/or homicide, work-related injuries/death, other injuries, financial problems, self-care, inadequate housing, and harm from others elicited by a person's behavior.

Table 10.1 illustrates the risk matrix that guides clinician thinking about the set of aforementioned risks and provides definitions and examples for each cell. The list of harms provided should be considered through the different lenses provided by each cell of the matrix. For instance, suicide is considered in terms of unintentional risk of harm to others, intentional risk of harm to others, as well as the obvious intentional risk to self. Work-related risks are considered through the lens of intentional risk to self, unintentional risk to self, intentional risk to others, and unintentional risk to others. The same consideration is given to each sphere of harm. We expand on the use of the approach in Chapter 11.

Table 10.2 is a clean version of the risk matrix without the definitions. This view makes it easier to appreciate the matrix's simplicity and for clinicians to commit the structure to memory and ultimately an automatic cognitive template.

Impaired Functioning: Critical Domains

Like assessment of risk, clinical attention to functioning is inconsistent. This is surprising because impaired function is a requirement for a *Diagnostic and Statistical Manual of Mental Disorders* (DSM) diagnosis. It is also significant that there is a lack of organized approaches to identifying and assessing functional impairment given that it accrues directly to risk.

Table 10.1 Risk Matrix with Definitions and Examples

Risk of Harm	Self	Others
Intended (consider acts of omission and commission)	*Definition*: Impact of the behavior is deliberate and volitional.	*Definition*: Material harm to others is deliberate and volitional.
	Example: Woman jumps in front of a subway train intending to be killed.	*Example*: A man stabs family doctor due to delusional belief that the doctor implanted a monitoring device in his body.
Unintended (consider acts of omission and commission)	*Definition*: Impact of the client behavior on themself is neither foreseen nor desired.	*Definition*: Material harm to others from the patient's behavior is neither foreseen nor desired.
	Example: Delusional woman stops drinking fluids due to belief that she is being poisoned.	*Example*: An intoxicated parent fails to notice his toddler enter the backyard swimming pool.
Iatrogenic (consider acts of omission and commission)	*Definition*: The adverse consequences of the medical intervention are neither foreseen nor desired.	*Definition*: The adverse consequences of the medical intervention are neither foreseen nor desired.
	Example: An elderly woman prescribed a benzodiazepine falls on her way to the bathroom during the night, suffering a subdural hematoma.	*Example*: A man started on quetiapine strikes a pedestrian while driving the next morning.

Table 10.2 Risk Matrix—Blank

Risk of Harm	Self	Others
Intended		
Unintended		
Iatrogenic		

As with the core elements of the risk matrix, the rationale of the selected spheres of function follows. The matrices of the approach are designed to inform one another. The identification of risks in the risk matrix is facilitated by the assessment of the client's ability to function in areas cued by the function matrix and vice versa. In this way, the matrices are interconnected and help frame the clinician's thinking about their client from three perspectives: risk of harm, ability to function, and symptoms. Areas of impaired functioning can also be viewed as antecedents to risks of harm and thus inform interventions and strategies to mitigate them.

Dependents

Children and others, such as impaired adults, elderly persons, and pets, are grouped here because of the similar responsibilities and tasks involved in caring for all dependents. The inability to safely and correctly perform such tasks is a core consideration. Remember that unintentional harm in this domain can result from errors or acts of omission. As we noted in the discussion relating to children in the risk matrix, unintentional harm from neglect accounts for most cases of child mistreatment. Core attachment needs such as love, physical and emotional nurturing, and security are thus included in this sphere of functioning.

Clinicians will usually be dependent on inferences to inform their suspicion that a client may not be providing adequate supervision or meeting their dependents' physical and basic psychological needs. Such suspicion may be corroborated by reliable sources or observed interactions with dependents (if present at a clinical visit). Difficulty with personal care increases the probability that clients are unable to adequately care for dependents and this therefore should be evaluated directly. This can require an appropriate community service being sent into the home and evaluating the client's ability to care for dependents.

Another aspect of functioning with respect to dependents is more subtle and especially related to children: the issue of children assuming a caregiving role for the impaired caregiver.

Housing

The primary concern related to housing is the ability to attain and maintain shelter. This includes basic maintenance, cleanliness, accumulation of possessions, and the ability to get along with neighbors. The ability to address hazards such as fire, electrical, and flooding is critical and has dire implications in apartment buildings. The timely payment of bills and rent is also critical because of its common association with loss of housing and homelessness.

The seriousness of impaired functioning in this domain warrants the use of objective assessments that provide a higher degree of certainty. This is because of the association between the experience of homelessness and higher rates of death, injury, and victimization. Direct observation of people functioning in their homes is critical, especially if they are the only adult or live alone.

Personal Care

This domain includes basic and instrumental activities of daily living (ADLs). Within this broad domain of personal care, it may be necessary to prioritize a person's ability to successfully manage their acute and chronic health conditions. This is particularly supported by the evidence that medical disorders, such as heart disease, disproportionately contribute to years of life lost in people with mental disorders.

The intent is not that the mental health clinician necessarily assess and monitor their client's other medical conditions. The mental health clinician's role is to review the client's ability to consistently execute the tasks required to care for self. The tasks we are concerned with are concrete. For example, in diabetes, the tasks to consider may include obtaining appropriate groceries, meal preparation, and adherence to the diabetic diet; monitoring, such as glucose self-monitoring; attending lab testing and other diabetes-related appointments; and other tasks related to treatment, such as medication adherence, behavioral interventions, and attending dietician appointments.

Considering sources of information, clinicians should obtain information with the greatest reliability and accuracy in reflecting the patient's health status. For instance, in diabetes and many other illnesses, to confirm the client's objective status, the clinician should obtain laboratory investigations or do so in coordination with others.

Work

This domain includes appropriate attendance and the ability to perform role-defined tasks safely and responsibly. We decided to separate work from education because of the extent to which work is associated with death and injury and the critical role that work plays in clients' ability to provide for themselves and their dependents. Mental disorders have a greater impact on the ability to obtain and consistently maintain employment than other medical illnesses. Periods of disability and employment gaps can further diminish clients' job prospects throughout the life span.

We make a distinction between employment status, level of attendance, and performance. If the person is currently not working nor looking for work, then there is no immediate concern for job-related risks. Employment status will have to be monitored, however, to avoid the client resuming work without the clinician's awareness and review of the roles, responsibilities, and nature of the work as part of a return-to-work plan. A clinician's awareness of risk of harm is critical in advising both client and employer/insurer on the timing and accommodations to optimize a safe return to work.

Licenses

Many licenses relate to activities with an inherent risk of harm to self or others and thus the need to demonstrate the skills required to safely function in the respective task. This domain is thus focused on the client's capacity to safely maintain personal and professional licensure and meet regulatory requirements. This includes those for motor vehicles and recreational vehicles; transportation licenses such as for trucks, trains, planes, ships, and boats; heavy equipment licenses such as for cranes, bulldozers, etc.; licenses for firearms; job-related licenses such as those for mechanics; and professional licenses such as those for nurses, psychologists, physicians, lawyers, and so on. Here again, the clinician will be dependent on information that is reported to them and usually limited to self-reports in the absence of information from others. This means that clinicians will be dependent on inferences based on symptoms and other domains of the client's ability to function. Even in the rare instances that clinicians may have an opportunity to observe a client's functioning in a licensed domain, the determination that a person is adequately functioning usually requires expertise in the said domain. As such, all that clinicians may be able to do beyond gathering self-reported information is suggest that the client request a formal assessment of their performance, especially in jobs for which inadequate performance carries a high risk of injury or death to self and others. Some jurisdictions have mandatory or permissible reporting for some licenses, thus enabling more robust risk mitigation. Otherwise, strategies available to the clinician will often be limited to engaging clients in considering potential risks to themselves and others, including their professional reputation. Many job-related licenses are critical to clients' sources of income, careers, and livelihoods, and a damaged reputation due to poor performance or an adverse event can have serious, long-term implications.

Interpersonal Relationships

This domain relates to the ability to maintain intact normative patterns of social interaction. The primary relationships we highlight in this domain are partners (romantic, sexual, marriage, etc.), families, workplace, neighbors, and strangers (including individuals with whom we repeatedly interact when executing instrumental ADLs). By far, the relationships that are most impacted by mental disorder and addictions are partners and other family members, followed by coworkers.

The range of impairments and scope of impact are enormous. These include eroding the quality of relationships leading to poor communication, aggression, low distress tolerance, alienation, isolation, and estrangement. Self-awareness and insight are also relevant to interpersonal relationships, and these impairments may be observable within the therapeutic relationship.

The interconnectedness between all the domains of functioning can be illustrated using key relationships. For instance, in romantic relationships, impaired ability to maintain personal hygiene, contribute to household tasks, limited emotional availability, struggle to maintain employment, and lack of desire to socialize are basic ADLs that erode or destroy the client's relationship with their partner.

Sexual function is frequently disrupted due to a mental disorder or its treatment. Although decreased libido and reduced sexual activity receive the most attention, it is important to assess for increased desire and activity or changes in sexual practices and their impact on partners. In addition, sexual behaviors can be associated with risks of harm to self or others by virtue of circumstances, injury, finances, criminal charges, lawsuits, or medical consequences such as infections.

Relationships in the workplace are considered because they often relate to concrete requirements of the job and the client's ability to adequately perform the tasks and to do so safely. Difficulties with frustration tolerance, anger, and violence are particularly important with respect to risk, as is a client's ability to respect others' privacy and personal space.

Education

This domain involves the ability to meet demands of educational endeavors (e.g., attendance, performance, and completion of tasks). Most mental disorders begin during the stage of life in which people are in school. It is a formative period that has an impact on future earning options as well as peer and partner relationships. Mental disorders can be devastating on a person's ability to meet educational requirements and goals across the life span.[6] Assessment includes attendance, completion of requirements, and performance, but it also addresses consistency in these and the degree of difficulty that the client experiences in completing tasks.

Accommodations for mental disorders have become widely available at all levels of education. These should not be viewed, however, as the end point in assisting clients with mental disorders. Such accommodations should be considered a reflection of the impairment related to the mental disorder and the need for improved treatment of the symptoms and impairments.

Finances

This domain focuses on the ability to manage day-to-day finances (paying bills and displaying good judgment in spending) relative to a person's discretionary income. Concern is about impairments that exceed the average financial foibles. To get a useful view of a person's functioning in this area requires obtaining detailed information about income and spending. Although uncomfortable for many, such a discussion is critical because of the impact of such impairment on housing, self-care, dependents, and desperate actions to attain money. The challenge of managing finances is greater the lower the socioeconomic status (SES) due to decreased discretionary income and minuscule margins for error. Mental disorders frequently have a devastating effect on obtaining and maintaining stable income, and they increase the probability that clients end up in a lower SES. In addition, clinicians need to explore for the possibility that patients with more severe illness are experiencing financial victimization.

Assessing finances objectively can be performed by reviewing the client's financial records either directly or by proxy. This idea may seem extreme or intrusive, but the consequences of financial impairment are more dire than those of many medical illnesses that are investigated using procedures that are more intrusive and uncomfortable. Mental health care needs to investigate functional impairments and risk with the same degree of seriousness.

Formal banking records do not ensure a complete view of financial management since clients may borrow money from friends, family, and dangerous lenders when judgment and insight are more severely impaired. To reiterate, irreducible uncertainty is inescapable in every aspect of our assessments.

Contrasting the Function Matrix to WHODAS 2.0

Although there are limited approaches to assessing functional impairment, there are several instruments in use. The World Health Organization Disability Assessment Schedule 2.0 (WHODAS 2.0) is one such instrument for quickly gathering information about a person's ability to function and has been promoted for use by DSM 5. It is transdiagnostic, atheoretical, and makes no assumptions about the cause of the impairment and thus is unaffected by comorbidities. Our approach's attention to impaired function reflects WHODAS 2.0's transdiagnostic and causal neutrality but is oriented toward mental disorders and addiction. WHODAS 2.0, although both thorough and efficient, does have some deficiencies related to mental health and addictions, particularly regarding risk. The self-report version is dependent on client insight, accuracy, and willingness to share their status and thus may be less accurate when the potential for harm is greatest. It does not explicitly address the ability to function in critical areas of high impact—for instance, driving, caregiving to children and other dependents, licenses, and housing. It does not probe a person's ability to perform tasks safely, instead focusing on ease, completeness, and time to task completion. It collapses both work and school and thus fails to consider the large differences in accountabilities, responsibilities, licenses, and overall risk of harm related to workplaces. Some of the other important limits of WHODAS 2.0 include the fact that respondents who have stopped working, attending school, or participating in society may select a lack of difficulty in these domains and thus fail to accurately reflect the severity of impairment in them.[7]

In contrast to the function matrix, WHODAS 2.0 attempts to categorize severity by providing clinicians with scores summarizing levels of impairment. The function matrix is focused on identifying areas of impairment that require intervention. Adopting the rationale that risk stratification is ineffective, the function matrix avoids it. The exclusive aim of the approach is to reduce harm and suffering. The approach takes a longitudinal view, drawing attention to aspects of the person's presentation that would benefit from intervention in order to reduce the probability that impaired functioning will accrue to harm. As discussed previously, categorization of severity is error-prone. It may lead clinicians to ignore impairments that are not categorized as severe at a moment in time and fail to reflect the ever-changing nature and complexity of mental disorders.

To be clear, we are proponents of WHODAS 2.0 because it has been widely trialed and used. We are not suggesting that our approach replace it but, rather, that the function matrix has a greater focus on impairments that can accrue to harm relevant to mental disorders.

The Function Matrix Categories: Observed, Reported, and Suspected

The structure of the function matrix also alerts the clinician to the degree of confidence they should have in the information informing their impression. This is facilitated by guiding the explicit consideration of the data's source using observed, reported, and suspected categories. Generally, direct observations and measures of a person's ability to function warrant greater confidence in the accuracy of an impression than uncorroborated reports from the patient or others, which in turn warrant more confidence than the clinician's suspicions. Clinical suspicions, however, can easily be confused as facts when clinicians are in the midst of conducting assessments. Overconfidence in our intuition and gut feelings can intensify this illusion.

Unless the clinician has had the opportunity to directly observe or hear from those qualified to directly assess the client's functioning, the clinician is advised to maintain very low levels of confidence in their impressions. Effort should be made to gather informed and repeated observations of the client's functioning in their natural environment. Still, even the relative superiority of such information is permeated with uncertainty because it is inevitably episodic. We need to hold our impressions lightly and continuously revise them until remission is achieved.

The Function Matrix

Data that are collected about functioning are organized into three categories: observed, reported, and suspected. These categories serve a number of functions. One of which is to help elucidate the quality of the information upon which we base our judgments. For example, did we directly observe a person's performance in the workplace? Did someone tell us about it, or did we infer it? The categories also anticipate the long-term nature of mental disorders and the resultant movement of assessments across multiple providers and organizations assessing the same person over days, months, or years. Information in clinical records is often difficult to verify, and the person's condition changes over time. The three categories are intended to assist users of the clinical record by defining the source of the information and helping stratify the relative certainty of each data point. For instance, direct observation of performance is likely to be more accurate than what is reported, and in turn, what is reported should be considered more reliable than our suspicions. We elaborate on the importance of the category of *suspected* in the symptom matrix.

A broader systemic issue that is not well addressed in clinical practice but is made overt in the RFS approach is the necessity of consistently gathering corroborating information from sources beyond the client. This is captured by the *reported* cue/column in the matrices and includes reports from both the patient and others. This prompts the clinician to inquire into the observations of others starting with those closest to the client. Particularly in North America, preservation of autonomy and individual choice has primacy even when the person's judgment has been significantly eroded. Furthermore, we rarely consider collateral harm to those beyond the index case and ignore that they were given no choice in being harmed. The majority of people are treated in isolation. This stands out as contradictory to the stated concern that our environments are critical to our mental states and behaviors. Minimizing the importance of information from others is at odds with the impact of mental disorders on reducing a person's ability to provide accurate and complete information. Involving others also helps protect us from our certainty and arrogance and enables a more complete view of the person's functioning, environment, and potential risks. Therefore, within the context of practice and training, we need to emphasize the critical involvement of others on assessing and managing mental disorders over time. It is inevitable that when we have a cross-sectional view of an individual's condition, we will miss important information relative to risk assessment and management. What we are arguing is in direct contrast to our training's emphasis on patient confidentiality and the frequency with which we inflate legislated constraints as an excuse for not investing the time and effort to obtain corroborating information. Ultimately, this may result in abandonment of the client.

The domains of function we have included are as follows:

Personal care—basic and instrumental ADLs
Dependents—children, impaired adults, elderly persons, and pets
Licenses—the capacity to safely maintain personal and professional licensure (e.g., vehicles and machinery) and meet regulatory criteria
Relationships—the ability to maintain intact normative patterns of social interaction
Work—appropriate attendance and ability to perform role-defined tasks
Education—the ability to meet demands (e.g., attendance, performance, and completion of tasks)
Housing—the ability to keep and maintain one's shelter
Finances—competency regarding day-to-day finances (paying bills and displaying good judgment in spending)

Note that although some categories of function are the same as those in the risk matrix, the duplicate domains orient us to both potential impairments (e.g., ADLs) and how these may accrue to risk. The elements of the RFS approach are interrelated and are intended to overlap in order to reduce error.

Table 10.3 lists the domains of functioning and provides definitions and examples of information gathering in each of the observed, reported, and suspected categories. The table serves as a quick reference guide and overview of the foregoing discussion of each domain.

Table 10.3 Function Matrix with Definitions and Examples

Function	Observed	Reported	Suspected
Personal care	*Definition*: Basic ADLs witnessed by the physician or other clinician. Walking, maintaining continence, and managing money are the three that could be observed or directly assessed.	*Definition*: ADLs communicated by the person or others.	*Definition*: Clinician infers impaired personal care on the basis of indirect or absent information, or manner of response.
	Example: After the person leaves the exam room, the chair is wet and foul smelling.	*Example*: The person's husband reports that he assists her to dress.	*Example*: The person is poorly groomed and is malodorous.
Dependents	*Definition*: The clinician witnesses neglect or mistreatment of dependents.	*Definition*:Impaired ability to care for dependents is communicated by the person or others.	*Definition*: Clinician infers an impaired ability to care for dependents based on observed or reported phenomena.
	Example: During the assessment, a mother shows no response to her infant's cries.	*Example*: The person reports he has forgotten to pick up his son from school several times.	*Example*: The client states she begins drinking alcohol at 4 p.m. and by 8 p.m. has difficulty "controlling" the children.
Licenses	*Definition*: Witnessed behavior in direct violation of the conditions of licensure.	*Definition*: Violation of licensure or lack of fitness communicated to clinician by client or others.	*Definition*: Inferred from indirect evidence.
	Example: Client arrives at the clinic intoxicated and having driven there.	*Example*: Person reports numerous errors in the operation of a crane due to distractibility.	*Example*: Level of arousal and attentiveness is grossly impaired on mental status exam, prompting the clinician to suspect the client is impaired in her role as a bus driver.
Relationships	*Definition*: Witnessed impaired or inappropriate social interactions with providers or others.	*Definition*: Communicated by client or others.	*Definition*: Inferred from indirect evidence. Predominantly obtained from narratives or signs and symptoms.
	Example: The person comes to the visit with his sister. He yells and threatens her when she begins to describe the family's concerns.	*Example*: Staff report that the client was sitting very closely to and staring intensely at others in the waiting room.	*Example*: The client reveals that she has no friends, people hate her, and she feels lonely.

Continued

Table 10.3 *Continued*

Function	Observed	Reported	Suspected
Work	*Definition*: Impaired attendance, performance, or behavior.	*Definition*: Impaired attendance, performance, or behavior reported by patient or others.	*Definition*: Inferred from indirect evidence.
	Example: An occupational health physician is given a worker's performance record.	*Example*: The patient gives the physician a form from work requiring medical support for 9 sick days in the past 2 months.	*Example*: The person reports coworkers are lazy and rowdy, and he is getting tired of telling them to be quiet.
Education	*Definition*: Impaired attendance, performance, or behavior that the clinician has directly observed or been provided evaluations of.	*Definition*: Impaired attendance, performance, or behavior reported by patient or others.	*Definition*: Inferred from indirect evidence.
	Example: A university health physician is given a student's transcript.	*Example*: The student reports that they have not attended class for 2 weeks.	*Example*: A student asks you for a letter to extend the due date for an assignment.
Housing	*Definition*: A direct or delegated home visit that includes the state of cleanliness and maintenance.	*Definition*: Impaired ability to maintain the home in a safe and hygienic state that is reported by client or others.	*Definition*: Inferred from indirect evidence.
	Example: The clinician obtains a report from a home visit service describing that the toilet does not work, the bathtub is used as storage space, the home is profoundly malodourous, and rodent droppings have accumulated on most surfaces.	*Example*: The client describes conflict with her husband relating to her dismantling of several floors and walls in the house. The client explains that she was simply attempting to eradicate parasites.	*Example*: The person has frequently shared with the clinician conflicts with various neighbors regarding multiple complaints.
Finances	*Definition*: Spending patterns, debts, loss of income, or altered cognitive abilities to make financial decisions that are directly observed by the clinician or related formal evaluations provided by others to the clinician.	*Definition*: Spending patterns, debts, or changes in income reported by the patient or others.	*Definition*: Inferred from indirect evidence.
	Example: The client provides the clinician with comprehensive financial records.	*Example*: The client's wife reports that her husband has depleted half of their life savings in the past 4 months and that she has no indication of where the money went.	*Example*: The client describes a conflict with her mother about the amount of hair products that the client buys. The conflict is triggered by the mother refusing to lend the client more money.

ADLs, activities of daily living.

Table 10.4 Function Matrix—Blank

Function	Observed	Reported	Suspected
Personal care			
Dependents			
Licenses			
Relationships			
Work			
Education			
Housing			
Finances			

Table 10.4 is a clean version of the function matrix uncomplicated by the definitions and examples. It is in this form that the matrix can be incorporated as a cognitive template or a simplified matrix to refer to during and after client assessments.

The Symptom Matrix

The symptom matrix focuses on those *signs* and *symptoms* most relevant to risk and organizes these phenomenologically into cognitive, emotional, sensory, and behavioral domains. The intent is to reduce the tendency to miss critical phenomena because they didn't obviously relate to the clinician's diagnostic considerations or the overt presentation. Signs and symptoms in each domain are also categorized as *observed*, *reported*, or *suspected*. Suspicions are critical to perceiving mental health symptoms because of our inability to directly observe most phenomena and, thus, the reliance on other signs and symptoms to cue the clinician to the possibility of such phenomena. This is especially true when patients fail to report phenomena independent of their degree of ability to do so. For example, a patient may not directly report delusions or hallucinations, but the clinician may develop a suspicion that these symptoms are present based on inferences from other phenomena. From a human judgment perspective, it is critical to explicitly identify that clinicians make inferences about the presence of many symptoms and that these inferences are suspicions rather than fact. This encourages clinicians to avoid unwarranted certainty in their judgment and to continue to test their suspicions as hypotheses by gathering additional information over time.

The following are critical symptoms to consider:

- Suicidal thoughts
- Homicidal thoughts
- Hopelessness
- Command hallucinations
- Other hallucinations
- Delusions
- Grandiosity
- Anger
- Attention deficits
- Memory deficits
- Judgment
- Alcohol use
- Substance use
- Impaired insight
- Impulsivity

Although the most salient aspect of the approach is first and foremost risk, in practice, we begin by asking about the client's/patient's symptoms and signs. These provide us with information leading to function and risks and may often be more concordant with why the patient is seeking care. The symptom matrix can also assist in organizing the information we receive and elicit.

Table 10.5 provides details about the key symptoms attended to in the symptom matrix, including their relevance to the identification of risk. However, the explanations provided are limited to key reasons for including the symptom in the risk matrix and should not be considered as operational definitions of the symptoms.

In addition to the matrices, we have found the Venn diagram shown in Figure 10.1 to be extremely useful in clinical practice, whether during an initial assessment or for ongoing monitoring. It is a concise way to consider the RFS approach, particularly when the clinician is operating under extreme time pressure but wants to be sure that they do not miss these critical aspects of the person's presentation. Think of it as RFS on a page or as a memory aid.

Having described the RFS approach to risk identification, we demonstrate its use in greater detail by comparing it to practice as usual. Case examples illustrates how the approach can modify assessment and management.

Table 10.5 Symptoms Delineated

Category	Symptom	Explanation
Cognitive	Suicidal thoughts	Their identification is frequently missed, and when found, often anchors clinicians' thinking, inadvertently precluding the survey for the additional risks listed in Table 10.1.
	Homicidal thoughts	They occur more frequently than related behaviors but are often not asked about. They can lead to catastrophic events including multiple targets.
	Delusions	The priority is to focus on beliefs that relate to risk and compel the patient to act.
	Grandiosity	Exaggerated beliefs that one is not bound by physical, mental, or financial limits and the potential for these beliefs to lead to harm.
	Attention deficits	Often associated with unintended risk (e.g., motor vehicle accidents).
	Memory deficits	Often associated with unintended risk (e.g., fire).
	Impaired judgment	Cognitive faculty related to discernment of consequences. Can the patient make wise or rational decisions, especially when action is required? Can the patient assess and draw reasonable conclusions?
	Impaired insight	To what degree does the person believe they have a problem, condition, or illness? To what degree does the person appreciate their identified impairments and risks? Impaired insight amplifies risk of harm and impairment, impairs judgment and decisions (sound familiar?), and reduces the success of interventions that depend on the person's actions.
Emotional	Hopelessness	A symptom of depression that commonly occurs with suicidal and homicidal thoughts.
	Anger	Anger can impair reasoning and judgment, and it increases the propensity for reckless behavior. It increases the probability of physical violence and threats of violence. It increases the probability of exhibiting behavior that frightens others and can provoke others to anger.
Sensory	Command hallucinations	Risky, common, but often missed. The command nature of the hallucination can be subtle and easy to miss despite eliciting related hallucinations. The clinician focus should be on the content of the command and its association to risks identified in Table 10.1. They are a risk even when the content is discordant with patient wants or intent.
	Other hallucinations	Prioritize eliciting the content because it reveals the risks most clearly.

Continued

Table 10.5 *Continued*

Category	Symptom	Explanation
Behavioral	Alcohol use[a]	Massively increases probability of suicide, homicide, harm to children, and every other risk identified in Table 10.1.
	Substance use	Includes both prescription and nonprescription drugs.
	Impulsivity	Poorly operationalized or defined but nonetheless frequently concluded by clinicians. Furthermore, the identification of impulsivity is inconsistently interpreted by clinicians but frequently leads to errors of diagnosis and truncated risk assessment

[a]Separated from other substance use due to its legal and social acceptance and its massive contribution to harm and impairment.

Table 10.6 Symptom Matrix—Blank

Symptoms	Observed	Reported
Cognitive		
Emotional		
Sensory		
Behavioral		

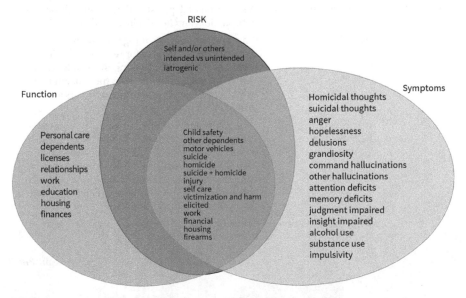

Figure 10.1 Critical risks, functions, and symptoms—at a glance.

RFS Approach and Usual Practice

To this point in the book, we have discussed concepts that relate to objective uncertainty, complexity, human judgment, fallibility, and other theoretical constructs that are not routinely translated into clinical practice. Although this book is an investigation and critique of mental health care, it is also meant to offer a way forward and to have a pragmatic application. It is intended to assist clinicians who are genuinely intent upon enhancing their expertise.

What follows is the use of a case, details changed to protect privacy, that was managed by one of the authors prior to the development of the approach. The case was selected because of the clear outcomes and the fact that these served as feedback to the author. As previously discussed, such feedback is rare in mental health care, and it was extremely valuable for determining how assessment and treatment failed. The case is then reviewed using a format that analyzes the clinician's actual approach and considers how the assessment and management of the case could have been modified by the application of the RFS approach.

We do not often have the opportunity to review our assessment and management approaches and compare them with alternatives. This is about broadening how we process what we are seeing, how we organize our thinking, and ultimately expanding our view of how to approach clinical practice.

Case Example: Actual Practice Without RFS

When I received the notification of the patient complaint from my regulatory college, I experienced the usual dread, followed by surprise, confusion, and frustration when I read the details. I recognized the complainant immediately. A 39-year-old, divorced female (G.S.) who had been referred to me by her family physician at the prompting of the patient's insurance company and trade union.

The complaint was made by the patient after a mandatory referral to child protection services. Failure to make a report can result in a conviction and fine of up to $5,000, as well as disciplinary action by regulatory colleges. (In many U.S. states, the failure to report can include being charged with a felony and the risk of jail terms.) In theory, such legislated mandates also protect clinicians from regulatory complaints or civil actions relating to their reports. The patient's complaint was accepted by the regulatory college because it did not cite the report to child protection services as the grievance.

G.S. was a primary schoolteacher who had been on "stress leave" for 1½ years. The insurance company paying her disability income was threatening to stop payments in the absence of a diagnosis beyond stress (stress is not a DSM diagnosis and is not usually recognized by insurance companies). The referral was from G.S.'s family physician and was not for an independent medical exam but, rather, for standard assessment and management. The patient reluctantly complied with the mental health assessment when informed by her union that it was unable to advocate on her behalf without a specialist's assessment. The client was already in an acrimonious divorce, including a custody battle for her 9-year-old child, and she was struggling to pay the legal fees. She could not afford to lose her disability payment or start another legal dispute.

At the time of the initial assessment, the patient was a reluctant historian and expressed her concern that a psychological assessment would compromise her career as a teacher and be used by her ex-husband to support his position in the custody battle. However, she agreed to proceed and to allow me to obtain corroborating information from her mother and workplace.

Over the course of three separate visits, the mental status revealed a thin, marginally groomed Caucasian female who was a difficult historian due to circumstantiality in her communication, contradictory information, frequent episodes of frustration and crying, and anger at me directly about the assessment. Her past psychiatric history included attention deficit disorder diagnosed at age 15 years, an episode of depression while obtaining her university degree in her 20s, and panic disorder while in teacher's college. While the patient and her mother minimized current symptoms and asserted intact functioning in all domains, the presentation was concerning though diagnostically ambiguous. The diagnostic impression settled on a probable recurrent major depressive episode of moderate severity, with a differential diagnosis that included adjustment disorder, malingering (although I did not add this to my consult note due to concern of it biasing the insurance company), major depressive disorder with psychotic features, bipolar affective disorder, eating disorder, panic disorder with agoraphobia, attention deficit disorder, and a concern about misuse of nonprescription hypnotics (antihistamines and diphenhydramine). In addition, I was concerned about the patient's lack of insight into her symptoms and that her judgment was difficult to understand in some domains. The patient denied any features relating to intentional risk to self, her daughter, or others, and the information from the patient's mother did not warrant concern for the child's well-being.

The patient disagreed with the differential diagnosis even though, as a result of it, the insurance company accepted her claim and continued her disability payments. Although she minimized the potentially negative effects of the antihistamines and diphenhydramine on driving, she agreed to discontinue them. She had no concern about her driving despite acknowledging that her continuous, angry ruminations about her ex-husband frequently distracted her from other tasks. When I attempted to explore the latter, she described an excellent driving record and derisively asked if my mind ever wandered while driving.

After discussing treatment recommendations and options, the patient spurned pharmacotherapy and cognitive–behavioral therapy (CBT) and only agreed to solution-focused therapy under threat of her insurance company.

I submitted a report to child protection services 9 weeks into care. This was prompted by the information contained in a request from her lawyer that I prepare a letter to defend against several criminal charges. These related to a motor vehicle accident that occurred a week earlier. The essence of the request was to assist her legal defense in linking the stress of her divorce and custody battle to the client's behavior at the time of the motor vehicle accident. The patient allegedly drove through a red light and was hit by a vehicle traveling through the intersection on a green light. Her daughter was unbelted in the front seat and sustained a skull fracture, concussion, chest contusion, and dislocated shoulder. Charges included reckless driving, assault (the patient assaulted the driver of the other vehicle), failure to have her child in a seat belt, and several other charges. The concerns I had that informed the report to child protection services were the patient's failure to ensure her child's safety in the vehicle and her assaultive behavior at the accident scene.

Upon investigation, child protection services found a ramshackle apartment, the daughter was underweight, and disclosed issues of concern. The child was placed in the care of the patient's mother (the child's grandmother). The patient was furious that I made the report, although police services had also made a report to child protection services the day of the accident.

Core elements of the client's complaint to my regulatory college asserted inadequate treatment resulting in her impaired ability to perform ADLs and adequately care for her daughter. In addition, the patient filed a civil suit. She claimed that my inadequate treatment contributed to her motor vehicle accident. In addition, she claimed that I did not properly advise her of driving risks when using antihistamines and diphenhydramine.

I did not foresee all the harm stemming from a motor vehicle accident. I also did not expect the complaint to the regulatory college or the civil suit. I was shocked by the child protection services description of the home and the daughter's care. Although I suspected that the patient was struggling to function more than she and her mother acknowledged, I did not envision the severity. At any given moment and seen in isolation, the impairments were not severe. Over many months, however, the multiple impairments likely accrued. It is reasonable to argue that if the patient and her mother had provided an accurate history, I may have informed child protection services earlier and reduced the chance of the motor vehicle accident and its sequelae. However, it is possible that the patient and her mother were also victims of the insidious nature of the risks. In addition, if the patient was not in a custody battle, she may have been more forthcoming. These and similar challenges, however, are common in clinical practice and are part of the complexity and uncertainty that we usually neglect. Consequently, let us test how the same case, with all its challenges, might have been addressed differently if guided by the RFS approach.

Case Example: Using the RFS Approach

Immediately upon receiving the referral, the approach would have guided my thinking. The approach guides the reordering of priorities so that risk identification is primary and establishing a diagnosis or formulation is secondary. In the absence of the approach, aspects of the referral reinforced my automatic preoccupation with diagnostic clarification. The insurance company was dissatisfied with the explanation for the teacher's sick leave and was demanding a DSM diagnosis. The family physician's referral focused exclusively on the need for diagnostic clarification and simply listed the client's multiple stressors. The patient herself was focused on diagnosis, although her preoccupation was on avoiding one and arguing that she was appropriately stressed. Simultaneously, she repeatedly implored me to safeguard her insurance payments. The approach would have focused me on risk identification, reducing the distraction from competing demands.

Although the referral focused on diagnostic clarification, conducting the assessment was challenging. The patient reluctantly assented to the assessment; thus, rapport was difficult to establish. Her circumstantiality, contradictions, and argumentativeness impeded clarity of all aspects of the assessment. The patient's mother, although a clear communicator, simply endorsed the daughter's information, offering coherent explanations to account for inconsistencies. I was left confused by the information I was provided; it did not fit any recognizable pattern. The only alignment in the cacophony of demands was the expectation that I had to provide clarity of diagnosis and satisfy all stakeholders.

So emerged the overarching question in my mind: "What is going on here?" Off I went in search of the answer, with the smudge of possible malingering clouding my glasses. In contrast, the approach would have set me on a clear course of risk identification and reduced my preoccupation with the diagnostic ambiguity and the bias of potential malingering.

Once into the assessment and sifting through the information, the fact that my observations did not permit me to confirm the information reported by the patient and others would have reinforced the inherent lack of certainty. The approach would have reminded me that my direct observations of the patient warranted greater confidence than the reports from the patient and her mother. This in turn would have guided me to more actively pursue my suspicion about the severity of the patient's symptoms and ability to function. At minimum, I could have coordinated a home assessment. The presence of malingering in the differential diagnosis, however, attenuated my level of concern for real risks, further reducing my vigilance in confirming the client's ability to function. I was also compelled by the story of the client's struggle to manage limited finances in the context of a difficult divorce and custody battle. I failed to consider that improving her ability to function and mitigating risks, especially to her daughter, ultimately aligned with her wish for full custody—independent of her realization of this at the time.

Instead, I developed a working diagnosis and thorough differential and proceeded with the only intervention to which the client consented—an intervention that was inadequate even for the apparent severity of her condition prior to its full scope being revealed. Using the approach, the patient's choice to decline pharmacotherapy and CBT would not necessarily have suggested that I find the patient incapable to consent to treatment and force our recommendations. However, it would have led me to emphasize to the client that her symptoms and the differential diagnosis required interventions beyond solution-focused therapy. I would have regularly revisited my concerns and recommendations with her and impressed upon her the potential risks of harm to her. This orientation would have prompted me to more seriously consider her capacity to consent to treatment. It also would have informed my reports to the family physician. Alternatively, I could have informed the patient that solution-focused therapy was inadequate care for her and that I could not conscientiously provide it.

As clinicians, we are accountable for recommending treatments that address the patient needs arising from our assessments. Informed consent guarantees the patient the right to decline the offered options but does not impose a requirement that a clinician deliver a treatment that is not indicated. If a patient is not satisfied with the treatment options offered, the clinician can simply inform the patient that they are not prepared to provide a treatment with which they do not agree. The patient will then need to seek care elsewhere. However, this is a difficult process to follow in the context of a therapeutic relationship in which the clinician is compelled by the patient's story and wants to maintain rapport. As clinicians, we usually try to avoid conflict and causing our patients additional distress. All of these forces act as biases that disrupt our clarity of judgment and decision making, particularly as they relate to the unpleasant issues related to risk.

A focus on risk identification may have revealed a constellation of risks that amplified concerns about the patient's insight and judgment. More important, her clear reluctance to engage would have led me to pursue more aggressive clarification of her ability to function in ADLs. Making my observations of her consistently poor grooming salient would have increased my suspicions of impaired personal care. This, in turn, would have increased my suspicion that she was impaired in her ability to care for her child, despite the mother's and client's contrary assertions. If I had been able to separate my suspicion of possible malingering from her 1½-year absence from work, I would not have second-guessed the degree of impairment that was emerging. I could have requested that the insurance company contract an occupational therapist to conduct a home assessment. I could have requested other sources of corroborating information. This would have included clarifying with her family physician and employer if the patient's degree of disorganized communication and argumentativeness were normal. Similarly, I could have clarified if her grooming was a change from her usual appearance. I could have obtained information about the client's possible weight loss from her family physician. I would have been cued to all of these by the RFS approach.

Instead, I developed a specious causal explanation that many of the impairments could be due to the underlying attention deficit disorder. The approach would have reminded me that such an explanation is fraught with uncertainty and irrelevant to the impact of the behaviors. Consequently, the priority would have been assessing the impact of her disorganized communication, irritability, and anger. My suspicion that both the patient and her mother were withholding information would have led me to question assertions that the patient's daughter was being well cared for. Combined, the degree of uncertainty would have led to a conclusion that I could not rule out risk to the daughter without a direct assessment by child protection services during the initial assessment phase.

These actions may seem excessive, but when viewed through the lens of reducing harm associated with mental disorders, and the degree of error associated with standard methods of assessment, the actions are reasonable, required, and protective. We underestimate the probability of anomalous events and their irreversible devastation. In other areas of health care, we rarely question performing invasive investigations, even as part of screening and prevention—for instance, mammograms, colonoscopy, cystoscopy, and others. Identifying the risks of harm in mental disorders with equal urgency, and applying interventions to mitigate this harm, is a key aim of the approach. Risk here, has primacy over diagnosis.

With respect to the symptom matrix, the client presented the following symptoms of concern: impaired insight, poor judgment, attention deficits, and anger. My impressions of the client's poor insight and judgments inconsistent with her wishes, would have allowed me to see how these could result in harm if I had been thinking about risk. I would have used formal testing to gauge the patient's ability to sustain attention in the presence of distractions. The fact that my differential diagnosis included a possibility of psychotic features in conjunction with the patient's anger would have added to the urgency of increasing the reliability and objectivity of my assessment. The latter is also an example of how a broad differential diagnosis facilitates a transdiagnostic approach and contributes to risk identification.

Essentially, the approach would have guided me to prioritize risk identification and reflect on the degree of uncertainty inherent to my assessment. I would have to conclude that an impression based exclusively on information gathered in the confines of my office was insufficient to exclude key risks. This would have prompted more intensive methods of assessment using community resources, use of less biased corroborating sources of information, and use of formal cognitive testing. It would have resulted in a report to child protection services early and before the harm to the multiple parties involved in the motor vehicle accident. Instead, the patient's child suffered additional harm beyond the poor care, which added to the patient's own suffering and severely compromised the outlook in her custody battle. Her finances were worsened, her driver's license was suspended, her cost of motor vehicle insurance would increase, and the criminal charges might compromise the security of her career. It is little wonder that she chose to file a complaint and pursue a lawsuit in civil court. In contrast, the use of the RFS approach might have limited the harm that the patient suffered though not her anger at a report to child protection services. She may have still complained and pursued civil action. However, my management would have been more thorough, and the harm that she suffered and sought compensation for would have been a fraction of that related to the motor vehicle accident and its sequelae. The impact on me and others would certainly have been less than the actual outcome.

Summary

A shift to prioritizing harm reduction in mental health care should be supported by a comprehensive shift in mental health training for all related disciplines. It is critical to incorporate irreducible uncertainty and inevitable error as key concepts in assessment along with prioritizing risk identification. Teaching approaches that explicitly account for the limitations of our knowledge, our biases, automatic processing, and the probability of error inherent to mental health care are necessary to reduce the unwarranted overconfidence in our field. In Chapter 11, we explore issues related to training as well as innovative approaches that might better address uncertainty in the domain of mental health and addictions care.

References

1. Clark LA, Cuthbert B, Lewis-Fernandez R, Narrow WE, Reed GM. Three approaches to understanding and classifying mental disorder: ICD-11, DSM-5, and the National Institute of Mental Health's Research Domain Criteria (RDoC). *Psychol Sci Public Interest.* 2017;18(2):72–145.
2. National Academies of Sciences, Engineering, and Medicine. *Improving Diagnosis in Health Care.* National Academies Press; 2015.
3. Centre for Effective Practice. Keeping your patients safe: A guide to primary care management of mental health and addictions-related risks and functional impairments. https://cep.health/media/uploaded/CEP_AMH_Keeping_your_patients_safe_2017.pdf. Published 2017. Accessed February 22, 2021.
4. Arya D, Nicholls D. Identifying and communicating clinical risk. *Australas Psychiatry.* 2005;13(4):366–370.
5. Bouch J, Marshall JJ. Suicide risk: Structured professional judgement. *Adv Psychiatr Treat.* 2005;11(2):84–91.
6. Mojtabai R, Stuart EA, Hwang I, Eaton WW, Sampson N, Kessler RC. Long-term effects of mental disorders on educational attainment in the National Comorbidity Survey ten-year follow-up. *Soc Psychiatry Psychiatr Epidemiol.* 2015;50(10):1577–1591.
7. Konecky B, Meyer EC, Marx BP, Kimbrel NA, Morissette SB. Using the WHODAS 2.0 to assess functional disability associated with DSM-5 mental disorders. *Am J Psychiatry.* 2014;171(8):818–820.

11

Uncertainty as Teacher

Education, Training, and Practice

It is clear that clinician training in mental health care has failed to counter our vulnerability to overconfidence, error, and the recognition of objective uncertainty. Neither the problem of uncertainty nor strategies to reduce clinician overconfidence are new. These issues have appeared in various guises. Through the lens of assessment methods, Paul Meehl began writing about it in 1954 and continued to do so for decades.[1] We have, therefore, known this for 70 years, and yet there is no evidence that clinician training has been modified accordingly. In addition, the opportunity for clinicians to improve the alignment between their confidence and objective success is minimal because useful feedback on their performance is miniscule. In this chapter, we explore several means by which we might address these deficits. We highlight aspects of education, training, and practice that are impacted by irreducible uncertainty and our professions' intentional and unintentional minimization of its influence on providing mental health care. We touch on barriers such as lack of feedback and its impact on precluding the translation of experience into expertise. We consider changes in undergraduate education to avoid reinforcing unwarranted certainty. We also consider the dangers of overemphasizing our superiority and power differential based on knowledge. In addition, we address the importance of training metacognition whether by mindfulness or a combination of other strategies. Ultimately, we want to chart a course to develop systems that provide clinicians with immediate and consistent feedback throughout training and practice. This is in order to combat overconfidence in our performance and therapeutic inertia and, most important, reinforce the virtue of humility in our approaches.

The field of mental health is in its infancy, far from the threshold of eliminating objective uncertainty. Despite these limitations, research outcomes in mental health are applied to the treatment of millions. Mental health research is often performed without adequate examination of assumptions, principles, methods, and the generalizability of its findings. For instance, the specious assumption that *Diagnostic and Statistical Manual of Mental Disorders* diagnoses have validity has been conveniently accepted by most research and all treatment guidelines. While other areas of human health have reduced the mortality and morbidity associated with numerous illnesses, mental disorders have climbed to the unenviable top position of burden of illness worldwide.

Most important, there is a great mismatch between our understanding of mental disorders and the degree of certainty that is implicit within formal education and training. These fuel our human vulnerability to unwarranted certainty and cloud the signals suggesting the urgent need for greater evaluation of our methods and performance. It is essential that these issues are addressed at the level of clinical training and continuing education.

This opinion is in agreement with the view of many, and, it is one of the central tenets to reducing diagnostic error discussed in the National Academies of Sciences, Engineering, and Medicine's report, *Improving Diagnosis in Health Care*.[2] Graber et al., using the recommendations of the report have proposed several strategies for achieving this aim within medical training.[3] Within the context of medicine generally, these authors concluded that "there is a clear mandate to improve diagnostic safety training in health professions education" (p. 110).[3] Neither source is focused on mental health, but the issues related to unwarranted certainty and overconfidence are embedded in their suggestions and are equally, if not more, applicable to mental health care.

At a fundamental level, irreducible uncertainty, inevitable error, and the recognition of them should be made overt at all levels of training and used as the foundation on which evidence-based care is built. Without deeply appreciating the ubiquity of uncertainty in all that we do, evidence-based care is easier to ignore. Due to the strength of cognitive biases and the illusions they create, we do not know to what degree any change to training would improve outcomes. However, we do know that the current level of overconfidence undermines the reduction of clinician error at multiple levels. As Ely et al. write, "Physicians value superior recall and shoot-from-the-hip decisions more than mental crutches, reflective thought, or disciplined task performance" (p. 311).[4] This description reflects the ubiquitous dependence on heuristics in clinical judgment and concisely illustrates the embodiment of unwarranted certainty in clinical practice generally. It may be that the illusory nature of *knowing* offers clinicians comfort in the presence of otherwise terrifying uncertainty, but the resultant actions are, at times, relatively impetuous. Mental health clinicians must be trained to understand that fallibility is the norm and not the exception, rather than being trained to know and to be certain. At minimum, we could reinforce the dominance of uncertainty and discourage overconfidence. Currently, uncertainty expressed by clinicians in training is often viewed as equivalent to failure.

A lack of recognizing and accepting uncertainty seems to be correlated with poor communication, increased use of resources, and medical student distress, according to Tonelli and Upshur.[5] However, their opinion that intolerance of uncertainty drives increased use of testing is consistently disproved by direct experimentation. The most common finding is that unwarranted confidence in assessment reduces a clinician's pursuit of additional information, testing, and consultation. In addition, clinicians tend to be driven by confirmation bias; thus, when ordering tests, they select those that support their opinion rather than refute it. It is important to note that such literature is derived from clinical areas with widely available investigations, thus the concern about excess testing. Mental health care does not have the luxury of worrying about excess testing. The closest thing to objective testing we have is structured questionnaires and interviews, and these are grossly underutilized. It is the unwarranted confidence that clinicians have in their untethered and untested skills that is the problem.

It is important to recognize that the learning cultures in which we are primarily educated as clinicians are often distinct from those in which we practice. Both the authors were trained in an undergraduate problem-based learning program predominantly emphasizing formative self-assessment (developmental, open, flexible, and promoting meta-cognition) followed by a culture of mental health delivery that is summative (structured, standardized, and comparative measures). The performance criteria that constituted being a "good" student or clinician were different from and contingent upon the demands of each context. The discordance between these two environments may be worth addressing if we are going to change how we ultimately practice. It may be that methods of training that are problem-based are more suitable for dealing with the complexity and uncertainty inherent to mental health assessment. A systematic review of such curricula indicated that those assessed through subjective and objective measures cope better with uncertainty, have a better appreciation of legal and ethical issues, show strong communication skills, and are self-directed with respect to ongoing learning.[6]

However, self-directed learning is significantly dependent on robust feedback about clinician performance and patient outcomes. Leaving aside, for the moment, the propensity for clinicians to ignore objective feedback and justify bad outcomes, feedback loops for practicing clinicians are rare. The ambiguity of feedback that we currently utilize makes it easy for clinicians to ignore or discount it.

Expertise—Does It Exist in Mental Health Practice?

Feedback is critical if we are to learn from experience over time and increase the quality of our performance and outcomes. Expertise, therefor, is dependent upon feedback that is consistent, unambiguous and accurate. This has been studied by several authors as it relates to psychotherapy and other occupations.[7,8] The evidence suggests that mental health clinicians (psychotherapists, psychiatrists, and psychologists) in training and in practice do not have access to predictable outcomes or receive enough quality feedback to ultimately be classified as expert.[8] Their skills and accuracy do not improve over time, and they are no better later in their careers than novice practitioners.

We are, however, acculturated to portray expertise. This is where confidence, authority, and the promise we can solve any problem have their greatest utility. Unfortunately, portraying expertise does not achieve meaningful outcomes with our clients.

We should not be too hard on ourselves, however, because as we have suggested, the degree of complexity inherent to mental health constrains the clarity of outcomes. Nonlinearity between an action and an outcome in a complex adaptive system reduces the availability and reliability of feedback that clinicians can use to calibrate their judgments and decisions. Shanteau illustrates this beautifully.[7] Using the theory of expert competence, Shanteau focuses on the relationship between the characteristics of the domain in which a professional operates and whether it is possible for the professional to learn from experience (i.e., develop expertise). He concludes that "the task characteristics determine whether it is possible for experts to behave competently or not" (p. 257).[7] He describes the characteristics that correlate with limited development of expertise as associated with complex adaptive systems. These include "changeable stimuli," "less predictable problems," "unique tasks," "feedback unavailable," "problem not decomposable," "decisions about behaviour," "experts disagree on stimuli," "subjective analysis only," and "decision aids are rare" (p. 259).[7] Psychiatrists and psychologists have been consistently found to lack true expertise.[8]

It is important to note that physicians and nurses may or may not exhibit expertise also depending on the characteristic of their specific domain. This means that providing mental health care does not necessarily equate with improved performance with years in practice and number of clients served. It also provides more reason to be suspicious of confidence and subjective certainty in ourselves and colleagues. Pragmatically, the finding that "poor performance in experts" is consistently associated with the absence of decision aids suggests their importance and that their use should be embedded in mental health training. Otherwise, clinicians will continue to view such aids as unnecessary and inferior to their own knowledge and skills.

Don Moore notes that "repeated self-delusion with repeated disappointment is hard to sustain because experience helps correct erroneous beliefs. Sustaining delusional confidence depends on not learning from experience" (p. 157).[9] Mental health clinicians do not have the benefit of feedback about outcomes that would help them learn from experience and thus are susceptible to "sustaining delusional confidence" discussed by Moore. Without continuous and unequivocal feedback, a professional has no reason, or guide, to alter their confidence. Although most pronounced in mental health, this is a key deficit throughout clinical medicine.

Another issue is whether clinicians believe the outcomes are due to their performance and especially whether they accept that there is room for them to improve. Accepting room for improvement in judgments and decision making is considerably easier and more likely if we replace the cult of certainty that permeates training with an attitude that aligns more closely to reality. Graber et al. make suggestions on how education might be leveraged to improve diagnosis.[3] One of these relates specifically to perspectives and attitudes as follows: "Acquire appropriate perspectives and attitudes (acknowledging complexity and uncertainty, incorporating the patient's values, understanding patient safety and diagnostic error concepts, etc.)" (p. 111).[3]

Yet another concern regarding assessing expertise and outcomes is that some outcomes are non-events and thus there is no feedback to the clinician. This is especially the case in the aim of preventing harm and adverse events. Success is actually a non-event. It is difficult to know *when* to conclude that a non-event occurred as a function of clinical care. To quote Moore again, "Those who avert disaster will always be unsung heroes. Their success is a non-event" (p. 149).[9]

Aside from overconfidence in decision making, when asked to self-assess, mental health clinicians clearly exhibit a positive bias, rating themselves "extremely highly" and none rating themselves as below average.[10] Clearly, we need to find approaches that help us develop a more balanced view of what we can be certain and of what we cannot. In addition, it is important that we evaluate our training methods and which of these, if any, could translate into better results for our clients as well as increasing expertise of clinicians as they progress throughout their careers.

So, in terms of how we approach the training and continuing education of healthcare providers, how we address uncertainty will be important. Tonelli and Upshur discuss uncertainty from a philosophical standpoint as it pertains to medical training with a focus on the moral (the *right* thing), metaphysical (meaning), and the epistemic (knowledge—as in, "Do I know enough?").[5] Others, as addressed in Chapter 1, discuss it in terms of its many sources and issues. In Han et al.'s taxonomy of uncertainty, they organize it into three broad sources, probability, ambiguity and complexity.[11] They also outline varieties of uncertainty categorized as scientific (related to the disease and data), practical or systemic (clinician competence, processes, and structures of the system), and personal (client relationships and meaning of illness). Graber and colleagues also discuss the need for the development of *adaptive* expertise as applied to training and the need to move beyond *routine* expertise.[3] The "beyond" involves teaching trainees to develop critical thinking, meta-cognition, mindfulness, awareness of biases and the development of "de-biasing" strategies, "positive transfer," creativity and promoting rationality as a means for making clinical decisions, and error management. All of this is a means for dealing with complexity and uncertainty within clinical practice (in this case, medicine—although generalizable to other disciplines) that include similar factors identified by Han and others, such as clinician demographic factors, clinician internal factors (stress, fatigue, cognitive load, etc.), cognitive factors (styles, rationality, and biases), environmental factors, and systemic aspects of the condition and patient issues. Whether addressed from a philosophical, ethical, concrete, or other standpoint, making the subjects of uncertainty and complexity salient in education will be important. The hope is that by providing trainees with cognitive frameworks and other skills to mitigate overconfidence, clinical error in practice can be reduced.

Making objective uncertainty explicit could also be facilitated by teaching trainees to bring attention to, and express, their level of confidence in their judgments and decisions. Their confidence could then be contrasted to the degree of inherent complexity and uncertainty of clinical cases. For example, using longitudinal case simulations could provide trainees with continual feedback regarding their performance with respect to error. These simulations could be designed to illustrate the range of potential judgments or decisions and the extent of the uncertainty present at various stages of a case's progress. This would require that education on assessment include the objective probability of error in our assessments generally and specifically aspects of assessment that matter most, such as risk of harm and impairment. Following up on a randomly selected number of real-life cases to assess for errors of omission and commission would be a way to address unwarranted confidence. This would give training curricula clearer objective targets that align with subjective signals to which clinicians have more consistent access. If we look for clinicians' subjective uncertainty as a lever to learning, we ignore the evidence that clinicians rarely experience this. Evidence reveals that clinicians can more easily and consistently connect with their subjective level of confidence, and this focus provides both teachers and the trainees with a clearer, more reliable target to reduce error in clinical care.

To shift the culture of overconfidence would require that all course materials, teachers, opinion leaders, guidelines, text-based resources, and other sources of information explicitly acknowledge objective uncertainty in their content and how this may translate into clinical error. Most clinical practice guidelines (CPGs) are beginning to do this. The extent, however, is limited to specifying categorical levels of evidence that support each recommendation, and it fails to delineate the transience of the guideline and the implication for clinical errors. The pragmatic importance of explicating the transience of recommendations is illustrated in the frequency of recommendation reversals in CPGs in even a single 10-year period.[12] When viewed from a broader historical perspective, our errors in mental health are grotesquely obvious, as illustrated in Anne Harrington's book, *Mind Fixers*.[13]

In our opinion, the following factors may promote overconfidence in professional training:

1. The implicit and explicit encouragement of prestige and power of the profession (specifically medicine and psychology), its privileges, hierarchy, and the specialness of its members
2. Acceptance into professional training programs as entry into a club that oversees its own members (professional governing bodies) and from which it is extremely difficult to be removed
3. The reinforced perception of clinicians as powerful and extremely knowledgeable, with such authority being backed by science—ironic, given that science spurns dogma
4. The power and status differential between provider and client
5. The dependence of the client on the provider for help and the implicit reliance on their knowledge and skills. These roles are fixed even when the client is part of the same profession. The sick role confers low status compared to providers in the system.

Strategies that exclusively depend on subjective awareness in attempts to improve clinicians' individual and collective performance are well known to fail in formal quality improvement efforts. At minimum, we should adopt clinical approaches that are less prone to perpetuating and amplifying clinician biases, such as those achieved through transdiagnostic approaches.

Awareness of Cognitive–Emotional Processes

So how might we address these issues in our education and begin a resocial-ization of practitioners in the field? There is a need to appreciate that falli-bility is not prevented by rote memorization of transient facts or idiosyncratic manipulation of unproven theories. One concrete way is to consistently in-form trainees about the specific frequency of error associated with each type of judgment and decision that they make, along with the sources of irreduc-ible uncertainty and cognitive errors that blind them to errors. The cognitive patterns that improve the efficiency of experienced clinicians simultaneously increase their vulnerability to judgment and decision errors. These include type 1 processing (rapid, "intuitive," and automatic), heuristics (shortcuts—the use of pattern recognition), and cognitive biases or errors (that skew or narrow thinking).[4]

Teaching trainees about these early on, implementing practices to identify them, and provide ongoing feedback would at least help clinicians appreciate the inefficiency of such approaches, thus demonstrating the need for adopting clinical methods and aids designed to save us from ourselves. To reiterate, the most useful intervention for mitigating overconfidence is ongoing feedback about actual outcomes. Unfortunately, the current availability of unequivocal patient outcomes that could be provided to mental health clinicians is close to nil. Consequently, we are left to rely on case material and vignettes. We suggest cases drawn from litigation and quality of care reviews to peak learners' atten-tion, especially in continuing professional development (CPD). Combining cases with small group, problem-based learning would facilitate the emer-gence and identification of unwarranted certainty, heuristics, and cognitive errors, enabling participants to experience these in real time or identifying situations in which these are likely to emerge. One could then examine their potential clinical effects on outcomes and have frank discussions around how to reduce these. Ideally, this would be woven into the fabric of all aspects of teaching, training, and practice.

Kolb and Fry's model of experiential learning could provide a framework for self-reflection and lived experience of how cognitive–emotional processes unfold and affect decision making. The model targets students but is appli-cable to clinicians who are faithful to their work as a *practice* for CPD. In Kolb and Fry's model, the student has a concrete experience and then engages in reflective observation abstract conceptualization, and active experimentation in integrating the learning into real life.[14] The student may come to recog-nize and attend to situations in which automatic cognitive biases might nor-mally be active, disrupting patterns that narrow thinking and impair clinical judgment. There is evidence that this form of learning has a positive effect with respect to student perception of learning as well as actual learning.[15] Other effectiveness studies, however, are mixed. Developmental timing of learning methods may be relevant. For example, Kirschner and colleagues note that direct instruction is often superior to minimal guidance except in situations in which the learner has a great deal of expertise or knowledge.[16] It may be important to delineate what is to be learned when applying a specific teaching method. For example, if we are speaking about enhancing self-reflection, then learning that promotes discovery may be vital versus the acquisition of information or a skill that is likely best learned through direct instruction. Last, we know from disciplines outside health care that the provision of regular feedback creates an iterative process whereby the learner can adjust their performance. Unfortunately, to reiterate, within the delivery of health care and mental health particularly, such feedback is rarely provided, and when it is provided, it is often dismissed.

For example, at a presentation on mood disorders facilitated by one of the authors, error rates in diagnosis were provided to the audience. It was clear that this evidence was met with deep skepticism and the view that the participants were the exception. As is common elsewhere, our prejudices are extremely difficult to overcome, and often, the more they are opposed, the more entrenched they become.

This suggests the need for an approach that uses a variety of learning methods to help the clinician experience their clinical impressions as hypotheses rather than *truths*. Holding the uncertainty inherent to our work in the foreground at all times appears to be essential. This aligns with the concept of *beginner's mind* from the mindfulness field that, in the clinical realm, would encourage openness and curiosity toward a client presentation.

Epstein developed a mindful approach in which the student–clinician works to enhance their reflective capacity when assessing patients, turning the lens of investigation on themselves to inquire into what they might be missing. He calls this a "method for mindfulness in medicine."[17] This method consists of eight variables to assist student clinicians to become more present and attentive to their clinical experience. These include *priming* (preparing for a client encounter with mindful attention and reporting on their own thoughts and emotions relevant to the encounter), *availability* (being attentive during the clinical encounter as well as reflecting on one's motivations, actions, and their effects), *reflective questions* (the teacher helps students develop their reflective capacity and enhance their recognition and tracking of their internal process as it relates to the clinical encounter), *active engagement* (frequent teacher contact/presence to observe and be observed by the student when in practice), *modeling* (thinking and talking out loud while engaged in clinical processes—that includes recognition/correction of errors), *practice* (disciplined repetitive attention on an object of focus or process), *praxis* (embodied knowledge in action), *assessment and confirmation* [inventories of mindfulness facets for students client assessment of student qualities (e.g., presence attentiveness)teacher assessment (e.g., curiosity) and student self-reflection].[17]

Another group has outlined "12 tips for thriving in the face of clinical uncertainty," directly applied to medical training.[18] Their suggestions are equally applicable to all mental health clinicians and students and could be developed as a protocol for the clinical encounter. These tips bring attention, inquiry, and investigation of the student's, supervisor's, and client's cognitive and emotional processing. They consist of the following for both students and those in practice, summarized here:

1. In the rare instances that uncertainty is subjectively experienced, recognizing the automatic discomfort that comes with it, including the associated thoughts, emotions, body sensations, and impulses to act

2. Identifying objective sources of uncertainty, using Han et al.'s taxonomy[11] or another cognitive aid to assess whether the uncertainty is irreducible or a gap in the clinician's knowledge, skills, and attitudes

3. Recognizing and addressing one's cognitive biases that may be operating: This could entail having a list on hand of those that most commonly affect the student's thinking about the task in which they are engaged.

4. Expecting and planning for uncertainty with a "safety net" as related to diagnosis and risk: The RFS framework, focused on disability and harm, provides such a net and is independent of diagnostic accuracy.

5. Obtaining support from colleagues through peer support and mentoring: The assumption of a correct answer to clinical questions is prevalent and interferes with our ability to tolerate uncertainty. Speaking with colleagues helps normalize both the uncertainty and our discomfort. A colleague's perspective on management plans to incorporate measurement and monitoring strategies that illuminate errors of judgment and decision as cases evolve is also of benefit.

For teachers:

6. Modeling and normalizing uncertainty and the acceptance of it: Don't be afraid to say "I don't know."

7. Supporting and enhancing curiosity as an antidote to certainty and a narrowed view: Invite such an attitude informally or through the use of specific tools.
8. Discussing the degree and type of uncertainty in a clinical situation and the cognitive biases that may be present
9. Teaching students about the presence of uncertainty in mental health from the beginning of their training, in the curricula and during clinical encounters

For clients:

10. Enhancing communication with clients by discussing uncertainty as it relates to their situation or condition: This communication informs and aligns with a definition of diagnostic accuracy, enhances the client–provider relationship, and is consistent with client-centered care. Pragmatically, it enhances informed consent, which is protective for both patient and clinician.
11. Collaborating with clients in decision making: Incorporating client values and desires can help reduce uncertainty and guide the direction of treatment, reduce provider anxiety, and increase client autonomy.
12. Increasing the valuing of uncertainty in systems to ensure that clients can receive care even without a diagnosis: Gheihman and coauthors animate the silence currently surrounding uncertainty in nosologies by writing, "Amidst the 87,000 ICD codes, there is none for 'I don't know.'"[18]

The integration of skills to develop an enhanced capacity for self-reflection into clinical training is in process. Hutchinson and Liben have developed and investigated a course for medical students that teaches mindfulness intended to help them prepare for clerkship, to prevent a decline in empathy, and to learn skills for self-care.[19] These are what we term subjective awareness skills and also may be useful for recognizing unwarranted confidence.

These approaches have not received rigorous study to assess their effect on the degree of calibration between clinician accuracy and confidence. They could, of course, apply to all areas of medicine and mental health, although we recognize that this is a complex and large endeavor. However, such approaches could be studied and applied to mental health training to teach students to enhance the examination and nature of their own experience and processing, during and after the clinical encounter.[20] In the area of mental health, this is not such a great leap. Students of psychotherapy are often expected to apply these models to themselves as part of their experiential learning. The problem is that, to date, this appears to have failed in reducing overconfidence. A critical factor to stimulating self-correction that is missing is continual feedback about performance throughout all stages of clinical practice. It seems that at least with respect to medical training, by not providing longitudinal feedback on performance and patient outcomes and "focusing only on theories, principles, and details, i.e., the 'facts,' physicians are trained to limit their potential learning and self-correction" (p. 13).[17]

A major challenge to utilizing approaches designed to increase awareness of our fallibility is our typical work environment. The resource scarcity and bureaucracy in this context emphasize the "expense" of each clinical encounter. The focus is on quantity of encounters rather than quality or effectiveness. System needs (e.g., funding issues and client numbers) often take priority over client needs. To be performed in a manner that alters behavior, the use of awareness, recognition, and reflection requires uninterrupted time.

One type of approach intended to reduce diagnostic and other errors utilizes structured approaches that direct attention to priorities or common errors of neglect. Such approaches serve more as cognitive cues or reminders and are less about turning a mindful lens on the clinician's thought process. These approaches of course need not be mutually exclusive and can support one another.

Such frameworks aimed at focusing attention include checklists primarily aimed at reducing errors of omission (e.g., failing to provide thiamine intravenously before treating an emaciated and unresponsive person with intravenous glucose) and attentional neglect (e.g., surgically removing the wrong kidney). Another that is broader in its reach and sequential in use is clinical problem analysis.[21] Other approaches are organized matrices or charts that assist in managing complexity, such as the RFS matrix that focuses on harm and impairment along with illuminating the nature of the information that the clinician uses. What follows is a description of a number of these frameworks that should be incorporated into training.

Checklists

Ely et al. have outlined several formal steps, using checklists, that the clinician can take to reduce diagnostic errors: "For diagnosis generic checklists could force a reflective check, and specific checklists could force consideration of 'must-not-miss diagnoses'" (p. 307).[4] A general checklist operationalizes actions and questions to increase self-reflection and is another way to examine a clinician's cognitive process during the assessment process. Croskerry and others have extensively outlined common heuristics and biases to which clinicians are prone.[22] Ely and colleagues have designed a checklist for assessment to mitigate these, as follows:

- Obtain your own complete medical history.
- Perform a focused and purposeful physical exam.
- Generate initial hypotheses and differentiate these with additional history, physical exam, and diagnostic tests.
- Pause to reflect—take a diagnostic "time-out."
  Was I comprehensive?
  Did I consider the inherent flaws of heuristic thinking?
  Was my judgment affected by any other bias?
  Do I need to make the diagnosis now, or can I wait?
  What is the worst-case scenario?
- Embark on a plan, but acknowledge uncertainty and ensure a pathway for follow-up. (p. 309)[4]

Specific checklists are made up of relevant differential diagnoses and "cognitive forcing statements" that provide the clinician with examinations or investigations and potential pitfalls to avoid for specific conditions. These approaches are centered around the diagnostic framework and pertain primarily to medical conditions for which objective testing is available. However, this process could be generalized to mental health care and adapted to transdiagnostic models. Checklists have been studied extensively. Their use in safety-sensitive occupations and health care has resulted in significant reductions in error and improved quality. Although the investigation of such approaches is still early, this does not negate the judgment and decision-making literature that robustly illustrates the urgency of mitigating the faulty nature of our cognitive processing in clinical care.

Clinical Problem Analysis

Clinical problem analysis provides yet another way to systematically engage in assessing complex clinical problems in which there is often comorbidity.[21] The five steps of this approach are as follows:

1. Gathering important patient data—expressed clearly in the chart
2. Accurate listing of "activating findings"—important clinical data—if not objective, clearly indicated

3. Comprehensive "list of patient problems" (justified not hypothesized)—common origin and/or consequence based
4. Differential diagnoses for all patient problems
5. Action plan—including further investigation and treatment

This approach to diagnosis is aimed at reducing medical error and decreasing the effect of cognitive biases. A common refrain (authors included) is that this may seem cumbersome and time-intensive, as if these were sufficient reasons to snub them. Time is a component that adds to the irreducibility of clinical uncertainty, but time is relative. The point is that time constraints limit the accuracy of our judgments and decisions and should be coupled with reduced confidence. What is often ignored in mental health care, however, is that most patients are in care for weeks, months, and years. We need to reassess statements about the time we can devote to comprehensive assessments by judging such assessments not by a watch but by a calendar. Premature closure of diagnostic assessment, often with very little information, may lead to differential diagnoses of poor quality and devastating consequences. We cannot emphasize this point enough to oppose the forces that continually compel us to be brief. It is therefore likely that the long-term gain of assessing such clients adequately is worth the time. We need to encourage perpetual and broad assessment to enhance our accuracy and effectiveness.

Transdiagnostic/Phenomenological Approaches

Transdiagnostic models of assessment and treatment may reduce the impact of errors relating to overly ambitious diagnostic narrowing that is currently the norm. Identifying all the possible diagnoses in a presentation and utilizing this *differential* differently, as a cluster of equally probable diagnoses, respects irreducible uncertainty and the likelihood of missing phenomena that require attention. This also reinforces the imperative for utilizing such differentials by giving them a more pragmatic function in treatment plans and ongoing assessment. Furthermore, it addresses the overprecision bias in our judgments.

Even if we had all available knowledge and data relevant to the client's presentation, the degree of complexity (the number of interacting components and variables) exceeds the limits of human information processing. This constraint imposed by complexity should be central to our training. In our view, the outcomes in mental health care that should be primary are reducing the full spectrum of associated harm including injuries, death, and disability. Doing so would also slow the flow of suffering. The gross limitations and fallibility of our current nosology, and its application in research and clinical care, strongly suggest that harm be considered independent of diagnostic frameworks. If mental health care continues to adhere to the clinical axiom that a diagnosis and formulation is the most critical and effective way to improve outcomes, we will be ignoring the evidence of diagnostic fallibility and failures of our current approaches.

Our current training and approaches to assessment of mental disorders are inadequately oriented toward material risks and disability. Existing transdiagnostic models also lack this focus. The RFS transdiagnostic approach is intended to fill this gap but requires more rigorous testing to determine if it will help consistently reduce harm and impairment. Nonetheless, its current utility lies in demonstrating the confluence of interacting risks, impairments, and symptoms that can accrue to numerous harms. These interactions are ignored by current risk assessments. Utilizing and developing transdiagnostic approaches to management aligns with broad evidence that current mental health training, across all disciplines, is failing patients and clinicians alike. These approaches should therefore be integrated into curricula to provide different ways to use our current nosology.

Pending the development of effective computer modeling, such as used in meteorological forecasts, comprehensive assessments (e.g., the Structured Clinical Interview for DSM), combining checklists, and approaches such as ours are necessary. These would mitigate the degree to which the complexity of mental health exceeds our cognitive abilities. These tools provide structure and act as a cognitive aid. They guide the clinician's attention to multiple variables using specific cues, whether in the form of questions (e.g., regarding clinician cognitive processing, client intention, or motivation), lists of phenomena, contexts, or diagnoses.

The acknowledgment of our fallibility in making judgments and decisions should be embraced as essential to our education as mental health clinicians. This means that we must be trained to be humble in the face of complexity and objective uncertainty and to remain mindful that we know very little about the antecedents to the disruptions of the mind. Rather than ask such questions of our trainees as "What are the causes of psychosis?" we might ask our students, "What might we be missing or not considering that is of critical importance?"—turning the lens to what we don't know rather than what we do know. This, of course, would require a change in values for clinicians, orienting them toward a curious and open stance rather than one of certainty and overconfidence. Ironically, this includes a shift in mental health training toward the valuing and consistent use of inventories, checklists, and matrices, as well as other comprehensive assessments. It may seem contradictory to espouse an acceptance of complexity and uncertainty and then suggest structured approaches to mental health care. The important difference is where we believe we have the greatest need for structure. The emphasis is shifted from using structures designed to strip nature of its complexity to using structures that support our minds' limitations in managing nature's complexity and the irreducible uncertainty that emerges from it.

The decision-making and judgment literature that opine on the multiple variables that clinicians and trainees need to consider to reduce error and improve management in general medicine focuses predominantly on diagnosis. Whereas the multitude of issues and strategies such as mindfulness, metacognition, awareness of cognitive biases, communication skills, and so on are useful for decentering from a perspective, our views and biases are automatic, entrenched, and extremely difficult to overcome. This applies to medicine in general and mental health care. It is virtually impossible for us to be free from the conditions and contexts in which we find ourselves and to take in all the information available, particularly in mental health.

The bottom line is that we clinicians believe that we are superior in our decision-making and diagnostic skills relative to cognitive aids or technological systems. The reality is that we are not. In the words of Marois and Ivanoff describing the brain's limits in processing information, "Yet, for all our neurocomputational sophistication and processing power, we can barely attend to more than one object at a time, and we can hardly perform two tasks at once" (p. 296).[23] This is probably a factor in counterintuitive findings that increasing data beyond a certain point is associated with deteriorating judgment and decisions accuracy. Computer modeling and artificial intelligence will eventually allow us to synthesize all the available client data for treatment and decision making. Until then, we need to learn from other areas of medicine and other occupations to consistently use checklists and other structured approaches that are helpful and underutilized. Systems that incorporate forcing functions are also useful to ensure clinician accountability and preclude clinicians from acting on judgments based on incomplete data and flawed thinking. Finally, building in ongoing feedback for trainees and clinicians regarding the consequences of their decisions is paramount.

This of course means a profound shift in training as it applies to both how we should be delivering care and how we should think about ourselves as care providers—we provide care but should not actually be the final arbiters of decision making. To this end, we agree with those who are calling for the use of automated systems to assist us.

Summary

Identification and exploration of the inherent uncertainty and ubiquitous error that exist within the field, as applied to both the training of mental health clinicians and the ongoing delivery of care, are essential. Without the integration of processes and formal tools to do just that, we do not see how we will decrease error and missed opportunities that arise from ignoring irreducible uncertainty and promoting overconfidence.

Returning to a comparison of mental health care with meteorology, what ultimately led to increased accuracy in weather prediction was the development of information processing systems that could handle the massive data. Before computer modeling, the more data human forecasters were given, the worse their predictions. In contrast, the more data provided to the computer model, the more accurate the predictions. As complex as weather systems are, so too is the human brain, the emergent mind, and human behavior. The information necessary to understanding changes to these is larger than a human being can process on their own. Thus, we must depend on structured and data-driven approaches to the assessment of mental disorders. Until we have such approaches and the appropriate measures, it is unlikely that improvement in mental health assessment and management will occur to any great degree. Drawing from Korean Zen, We think it is critical that, we shift from *know mind* to *don't know mind* and, Carol Dweck, from *wrong* to *not yet*. Given the amount of discourse on the subject of uncertainty in the literature and the increasing number of methods being proposed to manage it, we are hopeful that such attitudes will be embedded in the future training of mental health clinicians. This book is our contribution to the field, with its particular call to recognize the importance of comprehensively identifying risk and how this can help clinicians work with uncertainty to the benefit of all they serve.

References

1. Meehl PE. *Clinical vs. Statistical Prediction: A Theoretical Analysis and a Review of the Evidence*. University of Minnesota Press; 1954.
2. National Academies of Sciences, Engineering, and Medicine. *Improving Diagnosis in Health Care*. National Academies Press; 2015.
3. Graber ML, Rencic J, Rusz D, et al. Improving diagnosis by improving education: A policy brief on education in healthcare professions. *Diagnosis (Berl)*. 2018;5(3):107–118.
4. Ely JW, Graber ML, Croskerry P. Checklists to reduce diagnostic errors. *Acad Med*. 2011;86(3):307–313.
5. Tonelli MR, Upshur REG. A philosophical approach to addressing uncertainty in medical education. *Acad Med*. 2019;94(4):507–511.

6. Koh GC, Khoo HE, Wong ML, Koh D. The effects of problem-based learning during medical school on physician competency: A systematic review. *CMAJ.* 2008;178(1):34–41.

7. Shanteau J. Competence in experts: The role of task characteristics. *Organ Behav Hum Decis Process.* 1992;53(2):252–266.

8. Tracey TJG, Wampold BE, Lichtenberg JW, Goodyear RK. Expertise in psychotherapy: An elusive goal? *Am Psychol.* 2014;69(3):218–229.

9. Moore DA. *Perfectly Confident: How to Calibrate Your Decisions Wisely.* Kindle ed. Harper Business; 2020.

10. Walfish S, McAlister B, O'Donnell P, Lambert MJ. An investigation of self-assessment bias in mental health providers. *Psychol Rep.* 2012;110(2):639–644.

11. Han P, Klein W, Arora N. Varieties of uncertainty in health care: A conceptual taxonomy. *Med Decis Making.* 2011;31(6):828–838.

12. Prasad V, Vandross A, Toomey C, et al. A decade of reversal: An analysis of 146 contradicted medical practices. *Mayo Clin Proc.* 2013;88(8):790–798.

13. Harrington A. *Mind Fixers: Psychiatry's Troubled Search for the Biology of Mental Illness.* Norton; 2019.

14. Kolb D, Fry R. Toward an applied theory of experiential learning. In: Cooper C, ed. *Theories of Group Process.* Wiley; 1975:33–57.

15. Burch G, Batchelor J, Heller N, Shaw J, Kendall W, Turner B. Experiential learning—What do we know? A meta-analysis of 40 years of research. *Dev Business Simulation Experiential Learning.* 2014;41:279–283.

16. Kirschner PA, Sweller J, Clark RE. Why minimal guidance during instruction does not work: An analysis of the failure of constructivist, discovery, problem-based, experiential, and inquiry-based teaching. *Educ Psychologist.* 2006;41(2):75–86.

17. Epstein RM. Mindful practice in action (II): Cultivating habits of mind. *Families Systems Health.* 2003;21(1):11–17.

18. Gheihman G, Johnson M, Simpkin AL. Twelve tips for thriving in the face of clinical uncertainty. *Med Teach.* 2020;42(5):493–499.

19. Hutchinson TA, Liben S. Mindful medical practice: An innovative core course to prepare medical students for clerkship. *Perspect Med Educ.* 2020;9(4):256–259.

20. Epstein RM. Mindfulness in medical education: Coming of age. *Perspect Med Educ.* 2020;9(4):197–198.

21. Custers EJ, Stuyt PM, De Vries Robbé PF. Clinical problem analysis (CPA): A systematic approach to teaching complex medical problem solving. *Acad Med.* 2000;75(3):291–297.

22. Croskerry P. A universal model of diagnostic reasoning. *Acad Med.* 2009;84(8):1022–1028.

23. Marois R, Ivanoff J. Capacity limits of information processing in the brain. *Trends Cogn Sci.* 2005;9(6):296–305.

Appendices

Appendix 1 consists of blank versions of the risk, function, and symptom (RFS) matrices. These are cognitive aids for ease of use in clinical practice, in the care of mental health patients. Such patients may present in an undifferentiated manner with symptoms suggestive of a mental disorder, already have a diagnosis, or are medically ill and exhibiting symptoms of a mental health concern. Appendix 2 presents a Venn diagram that may be thought of as RFS at a glance. This versatile tool may be used to remind clinicians of the limited risks and relevant functional impairments and symptoms that may accrue to risk in any patient. It is meant to cue providers to the fact that relevant phenomena overlap and interact and also to focus the clinician's attention to all variables that may lead to harm of the patient or others. Last, Appendix 3 presents the Centre for Effective Practice's Keeping Your Patients Safe: A Guide to Primary Care Management of Mental Health and Addictions-related Risks and Functional Impairment tool. This tool was developed using the framework of the RFS approach for primary care providers. In order to satisfy the advisory committee, please note that risk has been stratified into low, medium, and high. Given the concern that this stratification may orient the clinician's attention away from risks considered low or medium, we are not in agreement with this decision.

The Risk, Function, and Symptom Matrices

Risk Matrix

Risk of Harm	Self	Others
Intended		
Unintended		
Iatrogenic		

Function Matrix

Function	Observed	Reported	Suspected
Personal care			
Dependents			
Licenses			
Relationships			
Work			
Education			
Housing			
Finances			

Symptom Matrix

Category	Symptom	Explanation
Cognitive		
Emotional		
Sensory		
Behavioral		

Risk at a Glance

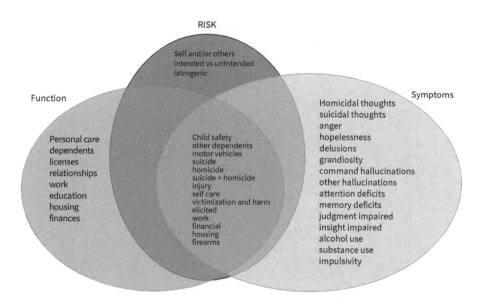

RISK

Self and/or others
intended vs unintended
iatrogenic

Function

Personal care
dependents
licenses
relationships
work
education
housing
finances

Child safety
other dependents
motor vehicles
suicide
homicide
suicide + homicide
injury
self care
victimization and harm
elicited
work
financial
housing
firearms

Symptoms

Homicidal thoughts
suicidal thoughts
anger
hopelessness
delusions
grandiosity
command hallucinations
other hallucinations
attention deficits
memory deficits
judgment impaired
insight impaired
alcohol use
substance use
impulsivity

Centre for Effective Practice—Keeping Your Patients Safe

A Guide to Primary Care Management of Mental Health and Addictions-Related Risks and Functional Impairments

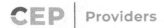 Providers

Keeping Your Patients Safe:
A Guide to Primary Care Management of Mental Health and
Addictions-related Risks and Functional Impairments

Introduction

Patients with mental disorders are often at high risk to themselves and others.[1,2] The purpose of this tool is to support primary care providers (family physicians and primary care nurse practitioners) in reducing harm in adult patients (18+) who exhibit signs, symptoms, or behaviours suggestive of a mental health condition. Considerations and resources are included in the tool to aid in decision making.

The objectives of this tool are to assist primary care providers (PCPs) to:

- Identify serious risks as a result of a patient's symptoms and behaviours
- Assess and intervene when a patient is at high probability of harming themself or others
- Reduce risk and manage immediate symptoms while diagnostic clarification is taking place

Table of Contents

The schematic below outlines the steps PCPs can take to reduce risk pending diagnostic clarification and ongoing management.

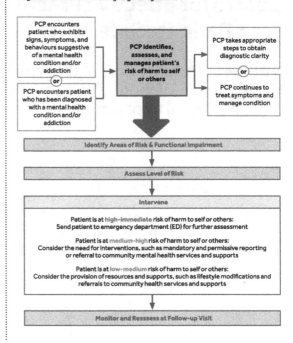

Section A: Exploring Symptoms and Functional Impairments to Identify Risk

Investigate the impact of a patient's symptoms and behaviours on their daily functioning (e.g. unsafe driving) to consider potential risks (e.g. harm to self or others).[3,4,5] With the patient's consent, include family and/or other caregivers as part of this discussion.

ASK: "How is your day-to-day life affected as a result of your [Insert patient's symptom/behaviour]?"

Consider the following domains in your assessment:[6]
- **Personal Care:** activities of daily living (e.g. cooking, cleaning, bathing, selecting appropriate attire, financial management, housekeeping, transportation, shopping, medication compliance) - **Dependents:** caring for children, impaired adults, elderly adults, pets - **Licenses:** driver's license, pilot's license, medical license, firearms license, law license, machine operator's license - **Relationships:** spouse or significant other, children, parents, colleagues, friends, community, medical team, substitute decision maker - **Work/Education:** appropriate attendance, ability to perform role-defined tasks, safety, completion of assignments

The following resources may be helpful to investigate the impact of a patient's symptoms and behaviours

- Assessing Functional Impairments:[7]
  This resource consists of two components:[7]
  - A list of signs, symptoms, and behaviours commonly associated with risk and functional impairment that if observed in the patient, triggers further exploration/investigation
  - A patient discussion aid to help PCPs investigate the impact on several functional domains.
- Sheehan Disability Scale:[8]
  A rapid, validated 10-point scale that assesses functional impairment in 3 key domains: work/school, social and family life.

Section B: Assessing Level of Risk and Identifying the Appropriate Intervention

The following section consists of two components: (I) weighing the risk and protective factors to identify and assess a patient's level of risk and (II) identifying the appropriate intervention.

──────────────── **PART I: WEIGH THE FACTORS** ────────────────

Use discussions† with the patient to identify factors that increase susceptibility to risk. Based on your assessment of warning signs, means and opportunities, determine if protective factors mitigate the immediate risk of harm to self or others.

WARNING SIGNS AND RISKS

Examples of factors that increase susceptibility to risk:

- Social and familial risk situation and/or lack of support
- Financial uncertainty
- Domestic violence
- Recent stressful events
- Expressed hopelessness
- Recent suicidal/self-harm behaviour
- Family history of suicide

†Directly ask the patient and/or family members (with patient's consent) about the above warnings signs, as patients often do not verbalize their thoughts or intentions unprompted⁹

Consider any factors that increase risk potential (e.g. background, history, environment and/or circumstance)[3,6,7,8]

↓

Probe to understand opportunities / means to harm[9,10]

- What are the available means of suicide or of harm to self or others? (e.g. firearms license, access to weapons, medications, etc.)
- Are caregivers able to sufficiently monitor and protect this person from harming themselves or others?
- Are there vulnerable individuals in the person's environment who cannot protect themselves? (e.g. children, elderly, other dependents, etc.)

↓

Probe† to determine if there are warning signs indicative of risk of harm to self or others

Suicide[9]
- Is the patient expressing or having suicidal ideation, intent, or planning?
- Is there evidence of suicidal behaviours, poor judgment, or poor impulse control?
- Is there a history of suicidal or para-suicidal behaviour?

Self-Harm[2,9]
- Is the patient engaging in self-harm or is there evidence of self-harming behaviour?
- Is the patient verbalizing intent to self-harm?
- Does the patient have a history of self-harm behaviour?

Harm to others[9]
- Is the patient verbalizing or thinking about harm to others?
- Has the patient caused others to fear for their safety?
- Is the patient expressing intense anger towards or fear of others?
- Is the patient making physical gestures about hurting others?
- Has the patient caused physical harm to others?

↓

Probe to assess the presence and strength of protective factors

ASK:

1. What or who has prevented or stopped you from [insert risk] until now?

2. If [protective factor] is no longer present, what or who else could prevent or stop you from [insert risk]?

EXAMPLES OF PROTECTIVE FACTORS[3,5,7,10]

- Strong perceived relationships with loved ones (e.g. children, parents, partners, friends, pets, other dependents)
- Strong, positive social networks
- Belief systems with strong prohibitions related to the identified risk (e.g. strong religious affiliation with prohibition against homicide)
- Optimistic outlook, identification of future goals, responsibilities/duties to others (e.g. child-rearing)
- A reasonably safe and stable environment
- Employment
- Using or connected to community services

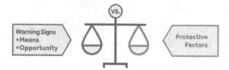

Warning Signs +Means +Opportunity   VS.   Protective Factors

Section B: Assessing Level of Risk and Identifying the Appropriate Intervention

---
PART II: IDENTIFY THE INTERVENTION

Based on your exploration of the risk and/or protective factors, assess the probability* and severity of adverse outcomes to identify the appropriate intervention using the matrix below. Determine the level of risk using scale below. Patients may cross risk levels – use clinical judgment to guide your assessment. See Section C for details on initiating appropriate interventions according to the level of risk.

		Severity of Adverse Outcomes		
		Non-Life-Threatening Functional Impairments (e.g. poor work/school attendance, poor financial management)	Critical Functional Impairments (e.g. serious injuries or health concerns, inability to perform responsibilities that impact the personal safety or health of others)	Life-Threatening Impairments (e.g. loss of life or limb)
		Increasing Severity →		
Likelihood of Occurrence *(Increasing Likelihood)*	**Incidental occurrence** (e.g. concerns arise indirectly from signs, symptoms or behaviours; differential diagnoses but no clear link to risk)	• **Implement direct interventions** (e.g. medications, psychologically-based interventions, or lifestyle modifications) • **Monitor over time** (e.g., book follow-up within next month)	• **Implement direct interventions** (e.g. medications, psychologically-based interventions, or lifestyle modifications) • **Refer to community supports** (e.g. support groups, crisis lines, and other health services) • **Close monitoring** (e.g. book a follow-up visit within two weeks)	• **Implement direct interventions** (e.g. medications, psychologically-based interventions, or lifestyle modifications) • **Consider mandatory and permissible reporting** • **Short-term monitoring** (e.g. book a follow-up visit within two weeks)
	Intermediate occurrence (e.g. recurrent behaviour exhibited likely to lead to events of concern; verbalizing intent to act)	• **Refer to community supports** (e.g. support groups, crisis lines, and other health services) • **Implement direct interventions** (e.g. medications, psychologically-based interventions, or lifestyle modifications) • **Short-term monitoring** (e.g. book a follow-up visit within two weeks)	• **Conduct mandatory and permissible reporting** • **Refer to community supports** (e.g. support groups, crisis lines, and other health services) • **Implement direct interventions** (e.g. medications, psychologically-based interventions, or lifestyle modifications) • **Short-term monitoring** (e.g. book a follow-up visit within two weeks)	• **Contact crisis support services** (where available) or ED consult (as appropriate) • **Conduct mandatory and permissible reporting** • **Implement direct interventions** (e.g. medications, psychologically-based interventions, or lifestyle modifications) • **Close monitoring** (e.g. book a follow-up visit within one week)
	Imminent occurrence (e.g. a related event has occurred; consistent behaviour exhibited; preparations for events of concern are underway; likely to lead to events of concern; command delusion or hallucination has been identified or suspected)	• **Refer to community supports** (e.g. support groups, crisis lines, and other health services) • **Implement direct interventions** (e.g. medications, psychologically-based interventions, or lifestyle modifications) • **Short-term monitoring** (e.g. book a follow-up visit within two weeks)	• **Contact crisis support services** (where available) or ED consult (as appropriate) • **Conduct mandatory and permissible reporting** • **Implement direct interventions** (e.g. medications, psychologically-based interventions, or lifestyle modifications) • **Close monitoring** (e.g. book a follow-up visit within one week)	• **Obtain ED consult** • **Conduct mandatory and permissible reporting** • **Close monitoring** (e.g. book a follow-up visit within one week)

Level of Risk

Low Risk	**Medium to High Risk**	**High-Immediate Risk**
Discuss lifestyle modifications, access to psychological tools and community supports	Initiate referrals to community supports and consider the need for mandatory and permissive reporting	Send patient to ED for further assessment

*The predictive 'risk for harm', as based on key signs and symptoms has yet to be validated: probe and use clinical judgment to guide your assessment. In situations of ambiguity or uncertainty, it is better to overestimate than underestimate the magnitude of risk.

Section C: Interventions

─────────── **HIGH-IMMEDIATE RISK** ───────────

Obtain ED Consult

A patient is at high-immediate risk of harm when life-threatening impairments (e.g. loss of life or limb) are imminent as a result of their actions/behaviours. These patients should be referred to the ED or local crisis support services for further assessment, where available and appropriate.

The intent of the following section is to assist PCPs in making key decisions, once it has been determined that a patient needs to be sent to the ED for further assessment. The aim is to reduce risks associated with transfers from community settings to hospital ED and to ensure that the level of risk is understood by the receiving ED.

If there are concerns that a patient may be a danger to you or your staff, do not prevent this patient from leaving your office. Allow patient to leave, immediately complete Form 1, and contact your local police to provide them with the completed Form 1.

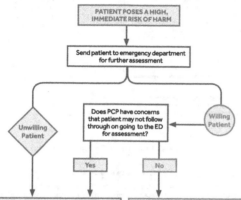

Tips for Completing a Brief Note to Accompany Your Patient to the ED

- Include the length of time that you have known the patient and examples of why this behaviour is atypical for your patient
- Explicitly state the adverse outcome of concern and your reasons for an emergent assessment
- Include PCP's contact information, and consider faxing note directly to the ED

Tips for Communicating with Your Patient

- "As a health care provider, I am committed to ensuring that your health and safety are a priority."
- "I am very concerned about your safety and I believe that you need to go to the emergency department immediately."
- "I appreciate that you may not agree with my decision and that it may cause you temporary discomfort; however, I truly believe that it will prevent you from long-term suffering and keep you safe."
- "Here is what I am going to do..."

Tips for Completing Form 1

- **Form 1** is used by a physician to legally bind a patient to undergo a psychiatric assessment, under the Mental Health Act (OHIP Billing code: K623 - $95)
- Neither the risk nor the mental health diagnosis need be certain; possibility is sufficient
- Physician can complete a Form 1 based on the information provided by others, as long as the patient has been examined in the past 7 days
- Complete either Box A or Box B, not both
- To increase the likelihood that the patient is admitted for assessment, be sure to stress risk and safety concerns

Please refer to examples of completed forms and additional documents for clarity: cep.health/mentalhealthrisk

① **NOTE:** Discharge planning plays a role in suicide prevention by ensuring ongoing support and care for the patient after an ED visit. PCPs can either be a part of the development of a discharge plan with the hospital, or can be included in the discharge plan as a point of contact for the patient to follow up with.

Complete a Form 1 if PCP has any concern that a patient will not go to the ED voluntarily.

Section C: Interventions

— MEDIUM TO HIGH-RISK —

Mandatory and Permissive Reporting

Patients' functioning in their daily lives may be affected by their symptoms and behaviours. The following section is intended to support providers to better understand functional impairments and assess whether intervention is needed.

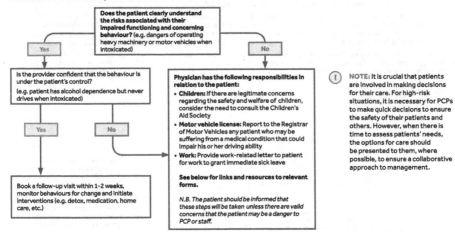

Does the patient clearly understand the risks associated with their impaired functioning and concerning behaviour? (e.g. dangers of operating heavy machinery or motor vehicles when intoxicated)

Yes → Is the provider confident that the behaviour is under the patient's control? (e.g. patient has alcohol dependence but never drives when intoxicated)

Yes / No

Book a follow-up visit within 1-2 weeks, monitor behaviours for change and initiate interventions (e.g. detox, medication, home care, etc.)

No → **Physician has the following responsibilities in relation to the patient:**

- **Children:** If there are legitimate concerns regarding the safety and welfare of children, consider the need to consult the Children's Aid Society
- **Motor vehicle license:** Report to the Registrar of Motor Vehicles any patient who may be suffering from a medical condition that could impair his or her driving ability
- **Work:** Provide work-related letter to patient for work to grant immediate sick leave

See below for links and resources to relevant forms.

N.B. The patient should be informed that these steps will be taken unless there are valid concerns that the patient may be a danger to PCP or staff.

NOTE: It is crucial that patients are involved in making decisions for their care. For high-risk situations, it is necessary for PCPs to make quick decisions to ensure the safety of their patients and others. However, when there is time to assess patients' needs, the options for care should be presented to them, where possible, to ensure a collaborative approach to management.

 The following resources may be helpful to providers with referrals to community mental health supports and services and patient management:

- **Mandatory and Permissive Reporting for Physicians:**

  - CPSO Policy Statement #6-12 Mandatory and Permissive Reporting[iv]
  The College of Physicians and Surgeons of Ontario (CPSO) have documented all instances of mandatory reporting (e.g. child abuse or neglect; impaired driving ability; safety related to pilots or air traffic controllers; railway workers and maritime workers; and occupational health and safety) and permissive reporting (e.g. disclosure to prevent harm) requirements.

- **Identifying Potential Workplace Hazard**

  - Contact the Ministry of Labour:[M]
  1-877-202-0008, option #3.
  Information will be forwarded to the investigation unit. It is important that the physician knows the employer and employment location of the patient to file a concern.

  - If a health provider is concerned that a patient could pose a potential hazard to themselves or to others in the workplace, the health provider is advised to contact the Ontario Ministry of Labour to file a concern. This can be done anonymously.

  **Providers must comply with the requirements, policies, and guidelines set out by their respective regulatory college regarding the completion of permissible reports and medical documents. Please see the following resources for more information:

    - The Canadian Medical Protection Agency's Medical-legal handbook for Physicians in Canada[xii]

    - CMPA/CNPS Joint Statement On Liability Protection For Nurse Practitioners And Physicians in Collaborative Practice[xiii]

- **Safety of Dependents & Family Members**

  - Reporting Child Abuse & Neglect: It's Your Duty[vi]
  Provides an overview of the professional responsibilities of health providers regarding the prevention of child abuse and neglect.

  - Contact your local children's aid society[vii]
  Healthcare providers are legally obligated to report suspected cases of child abuse or neglect to the Children's Aid Society.

  - The Advocacy Centre for the Elderly[viii]
  provides useful guidance on dealing with suspected or confirmed elder abuse or neglect.

  - The Ministry of the Attorney General[ix]
  provides an extensive list of options and resources for individuals who are being abused by their partners.

- **Reporting to the Ministry of Transportation**

  - Ministry of Transportation: Medical Condition Report[x]
  Physicians must report to the Registrar of Motor Vehicles any patient aged 16 years or older who may be suffering from a medical condition that could impair their driving ability according to the Highway Traffic Act (s. 203 and 204.).

  - The Canadian Medical Association[xi]
  Offers a guide to determine medical fitness to operate motor vehicles.

Section C: Interventions

───────────────────── MEDIUM TO HIGH-RISK ─────────────────────

Referral to Community Mental Health Supports and Services

PCPs can refer patients to several community-based mental health and addictions support organizations within Ontario, including supportive counselling, withdrawal management, crisis intervention, residential addictions treatment, early psychosis intervention, and vocational/employment programs.

ASK: When family/caregivers are known by the PCP to be included within a patient's circle of care, PCPs can ask if these individuals require additional support caring for the patient with mental health and addictions.

 NOTE: PCPs should ask patients about potential time and transportation barriers for the service to which they are being referred to. Additionally, when determining options for patients it is important to ask them about preferred language of service and take into consideration culturally appropriate care options.

 The following resources may be helpful to providers in accessing community mental health supports and services:

ConnexOntario[xii]

For a complete list of types of mental health and addictions services, visit ConnexOntario for a directory, operating hours and descriptions of local mental health, addictions, and problem gambling services.

ConnexOntario has helplines open 24/7:

☎ Mental health 1-800-531-2600
☎ Addictions 1-800-565-8603

Includes resources, such as 'Family Initiatives' that 'pertain to family groups participating in the planning and evaluation of care delivery, as well as the provision of services, such as self-help, peer support, education, advocacy, etc. These services can be helpful for family members supporting an individual with mental health and addictions concerns.

- **OCFP's Collaborative Mental Health Network**[xix] **(CMHN)**
The Collaborative Mental Health Network provides mentoring support and education to enhance the capacity of family physicians to provide comprehensive and quality care to patients with complex conditions involving mental illness or addictions.

- **Ontario Peer Development Initiative**[xvi]
Consumer/survivor initiatives and peer support organizations may be helpful for the recovery of patients.

- **ECHO Ontario Mental Health**[xvii]
ECHO Ontario Mental Health at CAMH and University of Toronto aims to help primary care providers build capacity in the treatment of mental health and addictions.

───────────────────── LOW-RISK ─────────────────────

Interventions for Lower Risk Patients

Immediate interventions can be provided pending diagnosis, such as symptom-specific pharmacotherapy, psychological intervention and environmental management. Discuss various options to develop a personalized plan that incorporates a patient's goals and values (i.e., preferred language of service and culturally appropriate care options). This section outlines considerations for symptom and risk management pending diagnosis.

Lifestyle Modifications[5,11,12]

- Work to develop management plan with patient
- Encourage a patient to actively participate in their own management planning
- Discuss protective factors and supports in patient's life and identify which protective factors can be fostered
- Encourage positive lifestyle changes, such as exercise, positive leisure time, and social engagement
- Offer advice on sleep hygiene and healthy eating as needed
- Discuss removal of risk-related items from the home (e.g. firearms, alcohol, unnecessary medications and poisons)
- If a patient is at risk for suicidal behaviour, work with them to develop a crisis and safety plan
  - Safety plan should include contact phone numbers for family/friends (emergency contacts), therapist contact information, and coping and problem solving skills that the person can perform independently
  - The Wellness Recovery Action Plan[xxiii](WRAP) provides supports and resources to assist a patient develop a crisis plan

Psychotherapy[13]

- Providers and their patient can initiate effective psychotherapy. Some online cognitive behavioural therapy treatments have been shown to be as, or more effective, than individual therapy with a live therapist.

Mood & Anxiety Disorders:

- MoodGYM[xviii] – Online Cognitive Behavioural Therapy
- Ecouch[xix] – Cognitive, behavioural and interpersonal therapies
- 211Ontario: Mental Health / Addictions[xx] – An online database of programs and resources in local communities
- Canadian Mental Health Association: Ontario Services & Support[xxi] – A listing of programs delivered by community agencies, hospitals or health clinics
- Centre for Mindfulness Studies[xxiv] – Provides mindfulness-based cognitive therapy, mindfulness-based stressed reduction, mindful self-compassion and specialized mindfulness training to the general public, healthcare providers and social service professionals
- Bounce Back[xxv] – A free skill-building program managed by the Canadian Mental Health Association (CMHA). It is designed to help adults and youth 15+ manage low mood, mild to moderate depression and anxiety, stress or worry. Delivered over the phone with a coach and through online videos
- See tips on How to use CBT with your Patients[xxii]

Section D: Ongoing Monitoring and Follow-up

Consider the following:
- Monitor and assess the patient's progress of care goals, clinical outcomes, satisfaction and unmet needs
- Liaise and manage care transitions or changes in care status to facilitate continuity of care (e.g. warm handoffs as patient transitions in and out of hospital and/or specialist care)
- Identify appropriate point of contact for the patient with respect to any care coordination issues
- Participate in multi-disciplinary case conferences to develop a care plan based on the patient's care goals. Additionally, with the patient's consent, maintain regular communication with hospital or community mental health and addictions services to foster an ongoing shared care relationship.

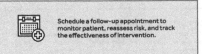

Schedule a follow-up appointment to monitor patient, reassess risk, and track the effectiveness of intervention.

Section E: Supporting Materials*

[i] **Supporting Document: Assessing Functional Impairments**
https://link.cep.health/amh31

[ii] **Sheehan Disability Scale**
https://link.cep.health/amh13

[iii] **Supporting Document: Tips for Completing Form 1**
cep.health/mentalhealthrisk

[iv] **CPSO Policy Statement #6-12: Mandatory and Permissive Reporting**
https://link.cep.health/amh12

[v] **Ministry of Labour: Reporting a Potential Workplace Hazard**
https://link.cep.health/amh28

[vi] **Reporting Child Abuse and Neglect: It's Your Duty**
https://link.cep.health/amh11

[vii] **Local Children's Aid Society locations**
https://link.cep.health/amh1

[viii] **Elder Abuse Guidance - The Advocacy Centre for the Elderly**
https://link.cep.health/amh5

[ix] **The Ministry of the Attorney General provides an extensive list of options and resources for individuals who are being abused by their partners.**
https://link.cep.health/amh24

[x] **Ministry of Transportation: Medical Condition Report**
https://link.cep.health/amh15

[xi] **Medical Fitness Guide - the Canadian Medical Association**
https://link.cep.health/amh21

[xii] **The Canadian Medical Protection Agency's Medical-legal handbook for Physicians in Canada**
https://link.cep.health/amh26

[xiii] **CMPA/CNPS Joint Statement On Liability Protection For Nurse Practitioners And Physicians In Collaborative Practice**
https://link.cep.health/amh27

[xiv] **ConnexOntario**
https://link.cep.health/amh19

[xv] **OCFP's Collaborative Mental Health Network (CMHN)**
https://link.cep.health/amh29

[xvi] **Ontario Peer Development Initiative**
https://link.cep.health/amh30

[xvii] **ECHO Ontario Mental Health**
https://link.cep.health/amh18

[xviii] **MoodGYM – online Cognitive Behavioural Therapy**
https://link.cep.health/amh23

[xix] **Ecouch – Cognitive, behavioural and interpersonal therapies**
https://link.cep.health/amh20

[xx] **211Ontario: Mental Health / Addictions**
https://link.cep.health/amh16

[xxi] **Canadian Mental Health Association: Ontario Services & Support**
https://link.cep.health/amh4

[xxii] **Supporting Document: How to use CBT with your patients**
cep.health/mentalhealthrisk

[xxiii] **Wellness Recovery Action Plan (WRAP)**
https://link.cep.health/amh22

[xxiv] **Bounce Back**
https://link.cep.health/amh17

[xxv] **Centre for Mindfulness Studies**
https://link.cep.health/amh32

*These supporting materials are hosted by external organizations, and as such the accuracy and accessibility of their links are not guaranteed. CEP will make every effort to keep these links up to date.

Section E: Supporting Materials*

Additional supporting materials and resources that may be useful for PCPs:

[xxvi] **Silveira J, Rockman P. Mental disorders, risks, and disability: Primary care needs a novel approach. Canadian Family Physician. 2016;62(12):958-960.**
https://link.cep.health/amh9

[xxvii] **Silveira J, Rockman P, Fulford C, Hunter J. Approach to risk identification in undifferentiated mental disorders. Canadian Family Physician. 2016;62(12):972-978.**
https://link.cep.health/amh10

[xxviii] **Form 1 – Application by Physician for Psychiatric Assessment**
https://link.cep.health/amh14

[xxix] **How to complete the Form 1 accurately**
https://link.cep.health/amh3

[xxx] **Form 2 – Order for Examination under Section 16**
https://link.cep.health/amh14

[xxxi] **Mental Health Act Forms**
https://link.cep.health/amh2

*These supporting materials are hosted by external organizations, and as such the accuracy and accessibility of their links are not guaranteed. CEP will make every effort to keep these links up to date.

References

[1] Silveira J, Rockman P. Mental disorders, risks, and disability: Primary care needs a novel approach. Canadian Family Physician. 2016;62(12):958-960.

[2] Silveira J, Rockman P, Fulford C, Hunter J. Approach to risk identification in undifferentiated mental disorders. Canadian Family Physician. 2016;62(12):972-978.

[3] Perlman CM, Neufeld E, Martin L, Goy M, Hirdes JP. Suicide Risk Assessment Inventory: A Resource Guide for Canadian Health Care Organizations. 2011. Toronto, ON: Ontario Hospital Association and Canadian Patient Safety Institute.

[4] Allan CL, Behrman S, Ebmeier KP. Primary care management of patients who self-harm. Practitioner. 2012;256(1751):19-22, 2-3.

[5] National Institute for Health and Clinical Excellence (NICE). Self-harm: longer-term management. London (UK): National Institute for Health and Clinical Excellence (NICE). 2011. (Clinical guideline:133).

[6] U.S. Preventive Services Task Force. Screening for suicide risk in adolescents, adults, and older adults in primary care: U.S. Preventive Services Task Force recommendation statement. Ann Intern Med. 2014;160(10):719-26.

[7] Centres for Disease Control and Prevention, National Centre for Injury Prevention and Control, Division of Violence Prevention. Child Abuse and Neglect: Risk and Protective Factors. [Internet]. 2016.

[8] Centres for Disease Control and Prevention, National Centre for Injury Prevention and Control, Division of Violence Prevention. Suicide: Risk and Protective Factors. [Internet]. 2015.

[9] DiGregorio RV, Green-Hernandez C, Holzemer SP. Primary Care, Second Edition: An Interprofessional Perspective. 2015. Springer Publishing Company, LLC.

[10] Centres for Disease Control and Prevention, National Centre for Injury Prevention and Control, Division of Violence Prevention. Sexual Violence: Risk and Protective Factors [Internet]. 2016.

[11] Centre for Addiction and Mental Health. The CAMH Suicide Prevention and Assessment Handbook. [Internet]. 2011.

[12] Durbin S, Ker K, Rawal S, Chan J, Ho A, Au Billie, Lofchy J. Psychiatry–Toronto Notes. 2009.

[13] Andrews G, Cuijpers P, Craske MG, McEvoy P, Titov N. Computer therapy for the anxiety and depressive disorders is effective, acceptable and practical health care: a meta-analysis. PloS ONE. 2010;5:e13196.

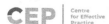
Developed by: **In collaboration with:**

  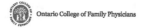

February 2017   cep.health/mentalhealthrisk   Page 8 of 8

Index